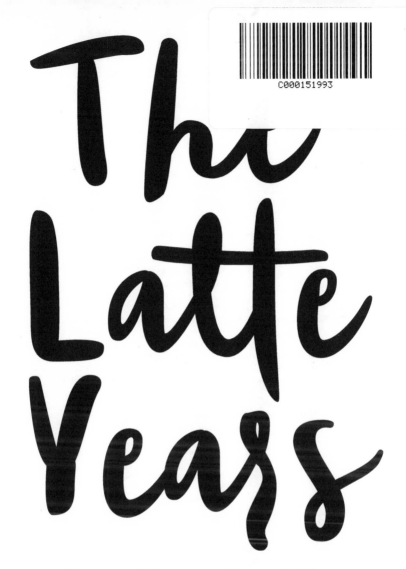

The Latte Years

A story of losses, gains and life
beyond the after photo

PHILIPPA MOORE

NERO

Published by Nero,
an imprint of Schwartz Publishing Pty Ltd
37–39 Langridge Street
Collingwood VIC 3066, Australia
enquiries@blackincbooks.com
www.nerobooks.com

National Library of Australia Cataloguing-in-Publication entry:
The latte years/Philippa Moore.
9781863957939 (paperback)
9781925203691 (ebook)
Moore, Philippa.
Self-actualisation (Psychology) in women.
Self-realisation in women.
Conduct of life.
158.1

Design and typesetting by Peter Long
Cover photo by Alice Gao Photography, Getty Images

The Latte Years

For my family, who have always believed in me.

CONTENTS

Prologue

*'Above all, be the heroine
of your life, not the victim.'*

NORA EPHRON

In April 2005, I was nearly twenty-four years old and weighed well over 100 kilograms. I got out of breath walking up stairs. My idea of a challenge was how to make a family block of chocolate last longer than an hour. I was married to the first man who had taken an interest in me. I spent most weekends watching DVDs on my own with the blinds shut and an entire cheesecake to hand. Clothes shopping was like going to the dentist – something I only did when I had to, and always painful. I had never left my hometown of Hobart, Tasmania – I didn't even have a passport. I'd never have admitted it out loud at the time, but I was bored, unhappy and genuinely didn't understand how life had ended up this way. I had been such a high achiever at school and university, the girl most likely, but I had reached my early twenties with no direction and no idea who I really was. I knew things had to change but life felt so messy and hopeless that I didn't know where to begin.

Now? I can't remember the last time I ate cheesecake.

It wasn't all about shifting some lard, however. Doing something about my weight and my health gave me the confidence to start tackling the other areas of my life that needed an overhaul, and it was then that the real work began. As the number on the scales went down, it became clear to me that I was actually in charge of my own life. I was the driver, not the passenger. But with that realisation came another – that my life as it was couldn't continue. And that was terrifying.

I wrote this book to answer the questions I had back then, in 2005 and 2006, and still had years later: what the hell do we do once we realise we can't keep sleepwalking through our lives? What do we do when we feel stuck? How do we keep going when we're afraid? What do we do when there are so many reasons to give up? How do we adjust to big, scary changes? How do we fight for our dreams when there's already *so much else* to do and a voice in our heads saying, 'Who do you think you are? Who are you to dare to want this? It's never going to happen.'

How?

You just *do*.

You write a book you're scared to write, the same way you train for a marathon you're not entirely sure you'll be able to run, the same way you build up the courage to leave a job or relationship that's not working any more. The way you decide to have a baby, move to another country, start therapy or do whatever is out of your comfort zone but closer to the life you want and the you you want to be. You get up every morning and you know what you need to do, so you do it. You fight your way up those hills. You feel fatigue soak into your bones and you get a stitch and you scream but you keep going. You have faith in yourself, because that is what faith is – showing up, every day, even when you can't see where you're headed.

Talking about it, worrying about it, wondering about it and thinking 'one day' is not how you do it. You just start. Anywhere. Because there is no other way.

It's not easy. And sometimes it doesn't work out the way you thought it would. But when you consider the alternative – staying where you are, changing nothing – I know personally that I would rather have tried. Mistakes are easier to live with than regrets. Every day you are choosing your life. Is it what you really want? More to the point, is it what you're willing to accept?

To be honest, a lot of the time that I've been writing this book has been spent trying to do anything other than write this book. I have spent many years trying to forget about some of the things I've written about. I had to feel my way through the chaos again, remembering being out there in what felt like a battlefield, where one day I was happy and excited about the changes on the horizon and the next it was an achievement just to get out of bed.

To write this book, I relied on blog entries and journals I kept at the time, consulted several of those involved and called upon my own flawed memory of this period in my life. I've taken occasional liberties with time by compressing or rearranging the chronology of some events, and left out unnecessary details, but it all happened. I've changed some names and identifying details for the usual reasons – I've also combined a few men I dated into one character to avoid being repetitive – but everyone in these pages is out there, somewhere. I know some of them will remember these events very differently to me. I've borne that in mind and tried hard to stick only to the memories and events that directly affected me and my story.

Why *The Latte Years*? I started a blog in 2005 called 'Skinny Latte', which was both my typical coffee order and a symbol, I felt, of the slim and sophisticated woman I desperately wanted to be. The blog found a large and appreciative worldwide audience, catapulting me to a different life and helping me find a voice, as well as some wonderful friendships. It would be fair to say that from the moment I hit 'publish' on the first Skinny Latte post, my life was never the same again.

I'm also a lover of literature, particularly T.S. Eliot, whose wonderful line about measuring out one's life in coffee spoons haunted me from the first time I read it as a teenager. I did feel, in many ways, that that was how I was living my life. Measuring it out in ordinary things, with not much room for spontaneity. Every day, and even every year, was the same. And the coffee? It was instant.

But enough with the coffee metaphors and on to the hard stuff.

I think many of us reach adulthood with multiple hang-ups from our early years, particularly about our own worthiness and whether or not we deserve to be happy. I was the same and have wrestled with the idea – and seen it similarly wrestled with in the media and in discussion of books like this one – that wanting a happy, authentic and meaningful life, when you already have so much compared with the vast majority of the world's people, is a bit selfish. That if your basic needs as a human being are covered, wanting more is a travesty. I'm not saying that I couldn't have done with a 'Seriously, don't you know how lucky you are?' tough-love chat at certain points in my life – far from it. I appreciate that the stories I'm going to tell you here are not exactly on par with fighting for world peace and curing disease. When I've witnessed loved ones face tragedies and injustices in their lives, it has indeed made me grateful for my relatively sheltered existence. Not a day has gone by since the events of this book took place, actually, that I haven't felt grateful for my life and the good things in it. But before that I didn't feel grateful for much at all. Far from feeling appreciation for my employment, my marriage, having a roof over my head and far more food than I needed, I felt deprived, resentful and guilty all the time. I was well aware things could be worse but that didn't make me feel better; it simply kept me stuck where I was and made me take that much longer to change things.

That's what I'm trying to explore here. We follow our heads, rather than our hearts, down certain paths in life, into careers and relationships; we are told constantly how good we've got it, and yet we're not entirely happy. We feel confused and guilty for feeling that way, which keeps us silent and trapped. This is a waste of our lives and does everyone a disservice. What are we here for if not to strive and to discover what makes us happy, what our purpose is, how we can best use our time and talents? It is not self-indulgent to ask those questions and go searching for the answers.

I also want to explain at the outset that this is not a diet book, nor a memoir entirely about losing weight – that is only part of my story. Weight loss was the tool that got me started and gave me the confidence and resources to start doing everything else. When the questions I'd longed to answer my whole life weren't being silenced with food and bad TV any more, everything changed. I realised I had the strength and the power to change anything I wasn't happy with. But I'm not saying that losing weight will automatically make you happy and your life will be perfect – far from it. In fact, within a month of reaching my goal weight, my life as I knew it fell spectacularly apart.

Rather, this is a book about changing your life and following your heart; about the complicated, messy ins and outs of trying to live the best, most authentic life you can. It's not about being perfect, but about finding a life that is perfect for you. I hope I can help you and inspire you, if you need that. At the very least, I hope I can make you laugh. A lot of it makes me laugh and fills me with affection for the people I knew and the Australia I lived in – a Melbourne that had Metcards instead of Mykis, a Hobart where Myer was still in Liverpool Street and MONA was just a Craig McLachlan song. The last time I came home for a visit I went to a newsagent and asked for a 45-cent stamp. The cashier gave me a strange look. 'It's 70 cents now, love,' he smiled. This is how time travellers must feel, I'm sure.

Mostly, what I hope I've written is the book I wish had been around for me ten years ago. A virtual arm around the shoulder, with a friendly voice saying, 'You know what? It's going to be okay. I've been there. I know how hard it is. But you will heal, you will get through it and everything will work out.'

On the other side of darkness, there is so much light. And excellent coffee.

So, pour yourself a cup. Let's get started.

PART ONE

Full-Fat Latte

*'If you want to do something, anything, with all
your heart, you can and will find a way.
But if you don't, you will simply find an excuse.'*

PAT FARMER AM

I'll start again on Monday

'Come on, do up, please God, just do up,' I hissed, the sharp teeth of the zip catching on my folds of meaty flesh, leaving angry red scratches, almost drawing blood. My internal organs felt bruised. My lungs ached from all the breath I had been holding in.

No wonder I had put off this shopping trip for so long.

After a year and a half of my thighs rubbing together like they were two stones trying to make fire, the crotch in my current pair of size 18 jeans had finally worn out. Even with flesh mushrooming out of the crotch holes, the jeans were now far too tight and I didn't have any others, apart from a pair of men's jeans in a size 40 (a more flattering fit, I told myself) and a pair of size 14s, my favourite high-school pair I'd kept all these years, hoping to fit back into

9

them one day. They would be considered vintage by the time I ever got my act together on the health and fitness front. These days I avoided clothes shopping and, on the few occasions each year I was brave enough to do it, bought whatever fitted me: tent-like stripy T-shirts, unflattering wrap cardigans and elastic-waisted skirts big enough to cover a trailer.

I had only brought into the changing room pairs of jeans in sizes I was prepared to accept I might be. There was a size 18 but also, in a fit of optimism after seeing how baggy they looked on the hanger, a 16. I had turned down seconds of dessert a few times lately so I was quietly hopeful.

The size 16 pair didn't even get past my knees. The 18s got over my bum but the zip refused to budge. I stood there, the fabric pulled tight across my flesh, the zip gaping open, feeling sick with shame. I couldn't keep fighting. They just didn't fit.

There had been many moments in my life like this. Eight years earlier, trying on the brand-new school uniform that had been bought for me several months before. Size 18. Too tight. 'We can't afford to buy you another uniform,' said my mother reasonably. 'You'll have to lose some weight.'

One month before my wedding day, three years earlier. My size 12 dress had finally arrived. I collected it from the shop, dizzy with excitement, and delivered it for safekeeping to my parents' house. 'Try it on! We can't wait to see it!' exclaimed my younger sisters. The skirt was full and glossy white but the embroidered bodice wouldn't do up. I cried and cried. 'You've got a month. I'm sure you can lose some weight. I'll help you,' my mother reassured me.

And now, 2005, a month away from turning twenty-four, here

I was, with size 18 jeans that wouldn't do up. 'You'll have to lose some weight,' I said to myself. '*Again.*'

Feeling tears streak my face and a horrible heaviness in my stomach, I finally conceded defeat. I pulled my black skirt with the elastic waistband back on and walked out of the tiny changing room that for the past ten minutes had felt more like an interrogation chamber.

I stalked past the racks of plus-size clothing – mostly hideous floral blouses and Winnie the Pooh jumpers that women my size supposedly wanted to wear – and headed to the photo lab to pick up two rolls of film I'd put in for developing after a recent long weekend away. I kept my head down. I hoped I wouldn't run into anyone I knew, as often happened in a city this small. I just wanted to be invisible. I felt ashamed, humiliated and utterly deflated, knowing that nothing I had done over the past eight years had worked. It was official – I was a failure. The idea of going on another diet, depriving myself of food when it was the only thing in my life that gave me any real pleasure, made me want to curl up in the soft furnishings section of Kmart and weep.

Eyes downcast, I nearly collided with another woman.

'Sorry!' I said, briefly looking up.

'Watch out!' she snapped, then added quietly, 'fat arse'.

By the time I realised what she'd said, she was gone. Much as I wanted to run after her and tell her off for being such a rude bitch, I didn't have the fight in me. And I *did* have a fat arse; I couldn't deny it. The tears came again but I was determined not to let them fall. I just wanted to get out of there.

I collected the photos from the lab and walked through the

shopping centre as quickly as possible so I could get to my car and get home, where I'd be safe from ridicule. I felt weighed down with the sadness and unfairness of everything that had happened in the past fifteen minutes. How could I make it go away? How could I make myself feel better?

As I walked I saw, out of the corner of my eye, the Donut King stand. The sweet, yeasty smell had my nostrils twitching. It was nearly closing time and I saw that their six-packs of cinnamon donuts were marked down to a dollar each. My husband, Glenn, was a big fan of donuts – well, any junk food really – so he would like those, I thought. I bought two six-packs and scampered out of the shopping centre to my car.

Sliding into the driver's seat, I put the bag of donuts and my handbag down on the passenger seat and retrieved the envelopes of photos from my bag. I usually dreaded getting photos developed but I thought I'd looked quite decent over the weekend in Melbourne. Pretty, even. I lifted the photos out and started leafing through them.

Oh. God.

My stomach dropped. I couldn't believe what I was seeing.

Glenn had snapped a picture of me in front of the giant, red-lipped, toothy-mouthed entrance to Luna Park; in it I was wearing a top that made my arms look like tree trunks. I had thought that tank top was flattering but it was actually very tight. There were visible fat rolls on either side of me, even with my arms rigid and solider-like against them, and my skirt looked more like a duvet cover. And my chin…s! How many of them were there?

A breath shuddered in and out of me and tears stung my eyes but I slapped the photo to the back and kept looking. Each photo

I saw made me feel sick and wretched inside. The thoughts that had temporarily subsided with the purchase of donuts were again on repeat in my head.

You need to lose some weight. You're a mess. You're an embarrassment. How could you let yourself go like this?

But then another thought entered my head, louder than the others.

This isn't who I really am.

*

Over the past few years my life had sunk to new levels of inertia and, as a result, I had got progressively bigger. After graduating, I had taken a stressful corporate job, and even though I went to my local gym every lunchtime, it wasn't enough to compensate for the comfort eating. To take my mind off how miserable I was at work I would scoff a packet of Tim Tams for morning tea and buy cans of Coke Zero and foot-long, mayonnaise-drenched subs on the way back from the gym. A couple of Kit Kats were permanently in my desk drawer in case of emergencies – and there were many of those.

And that was just what I did during the day. At night it was a whole other ball game. My husband worked similar hours to me but if he wasn't at work he was usually at a soccer or cricket game or club meeting, or engrossed in some kind of PlayStation game. We didn't spend an awful lot of quality time together. As for a social life, I hardly saw anyone apart from my family. Most of my friends had moved interstate, or I'd lost touch with them. Even my closest friend, Anne, was studying in Launceston, a few hours' drive away. To keep loneliness and boredom at bay, I turned to 4-litre tubs of ice-cream, packets upon packets of biscuits or blocks of chocolate in towering stacks. It therefore shouldn't have surprised me that the only effect the gym had had was to make my already worn-in size 18 and 20 clothes slightly looser. But feeling anything would have meant acknowledging how empty my life actually was. It was easier to eat.

Life hadn't always been this way but I found it hard to remember when I last felt truly motivated or energised by anything, or genuinely attractive – perhaps my wedding day, when I'd married Glenn, my first boyfriend, at the ripe old age of twenty. But by our first wedding anniversary, I had gone from a size 12–14 to a size 18–20, and stayed there. Life was busy and stressful as we settled into married life, which, I was disappointed to realise, just seemed to revolve around money and saving to buy a house, which meant having to stay in a job I hated.

And yet I watched other people my age finish their studies, as I had, and then set off on backpacking adventures or working holidays in far-off, more interesting places. I couldn't really accept or understand why I had missed out on all that. Wasn't life meant to be exciting and full of possibilities in your early twenties? Why did I feel like life had passed me by?

Just then, my phone beeped with a new text message – weirdly enough, from Anne.

I've joined Weight Watchers. Fed up with the fat party!!

I laughed but there were the tears again, stinging my eyes, my whole body flooded with hopelessness. Anne and I had talked about joining Weight Watchers the last time we met up but I honestly hadn't given it much thought since. I had no faith in myself to see anything through these days. I was used to having similar conversations with my friends, my workmates, my sisters and my mother, waiting for them to say, 'Oh, you're not fat! You're lovely just the way you are.' But when I banged on about needing to lose weight, no one ever seemed to disagree with me. Any discussions in this vein tended to trail off and my life continued to oscillate between weekend binges and *I'll start again on Monday* thoughts, a cycle I had been unable, or unwilling, to break.

I'd known Anne since we were sixteen and considered her as good as another sister. Her company lit me up from the inside. We both loved theatre and music, and dreamed of travelling the world. But, unlike me, Anne actually took action on her dreams and goals. Since we left school she'd worked various jobs that suited her vibrant personality – tour guiding, hospitality – and when she had enough money saved, she buggered off to wherever she pleased for however long she could afford. She always came back full of tales about her adventures. I was quite jealous, really. Not that I begrudged Anne her fun, of course. I just wished I was having some too.

I took a deep breath and texted back. *Well done, darl. Proud of you.*

The brutal truth was that Anne was smaller than me – and if she was joining Weight Watchers then where the hell did that leave me? I didn't want to be the fat friend. I didn't want to be left behind with the unhealthy habits – the sugar-loaded vodka drinks we drank like water, the packets of Doritos we went through with every movie we watched and the tubs of ice-cream (always low fat) we somehow always had room for. I didn't want to sabotage her either. It was just horribly inconvenient that my friend had decided to improve her life, because it shone a very bright light on my own.

Denial was becoming a harder and harder place to operate from. I was tired of feeling so uncomfortable in my own skin. But everything I wanted to do with my life just felt too hard. I was too far down this path now. For the past few years, as I'd grown bigger and bigger, I had wanted to bury myself under a rock, not engage with life or with anyone, and silence the voices in my head with food.

Speaking of which. I looked at the cinnamon donuts I'd just bought, the spicy sweet smell of them infusing the air, the oil they had been cooked in smearing the sides of the plastic box.

I have to do something. This isn't who I thought I would be. This isn't who I wanted to be. This wasn't supposed to be my life.

My throat trembled with a sob.

I put the photos and phone back in my handbag, then ripped open the plastic container of cinnamon donuts. I shoved one in my mouth and started the engine, feeling the yeasty sweetness billow into my mouth, crowding out all the thoughts.

I'd eaten three by the time I left the car park. *I'll start again on Monday,* I told myself.

Fat chance

When I think about my life prior to 2005, it's like I'm watching a movie about someone else. Someone with very bad dress sense (luckily it was Hobart in the 1990s and no one seemed to notice) and with no real sense of who she is or where she belongs. Someone brimming with dreams and plans, but no idea how to put any of it into practice. Someone who has no idea what a healthy relationship is – with people, with food or with herself. Someone who thinks if she is good all the time, and never rocks the boat, then everything will be okay.

This surprises me because even though Hobart, Tasmania, was still a pretty quiet and somewhat backwards place while I was growing up (you could still technically get thrown in jail for being gay, the most exotic shop in town was The Body Shop and, unlike most kids today, I didn't taste McDonald's until I was six), it wasn't as cut off from the rest of the planet as you might have thought. No, our news channels were full of things that were going on all over the world (even though a kid losing his teddy bear in one of Hobart's department stores did make the front page of the local newspaper once), and I was part of Generation Y. We were the children of astronauts, rock stars and political revolutionaries. We could do anything. We could change the world, if we wanted to.

My parents contributed to the feminist revolution by producing four daughters in five years ('Don't you have television in Tasmania?!' my uncle in Sydney joked when my mother announced her fourth pregnancy), all of whom wanted to take on the world in their own way. From a very early age, my natural talent was for bossiness (essential for the eldest child), but by the time I was a teenager, I had become so frightened of the world my natural talent seemed to be subservience. The only time the true me was able to shine was when I was pretending to be someone else. Hence, drama was my best subject at school. Playing a part was a place of safety for me. It was also something I was good at, something other people seemed to admire me for. Being one of four children who all loved attention, I craved admiration and relentlessly pursued it.

Until I was about eleven, I was one of those kids who was able to put away mountains of food and yet my body remained slender. I played lots of sport and I also had three younger sisters plus a tribe of friends in the neighbourhood to run around with. We were active kids, always riding our bikes, building cubbies and putting on plays. Unlike nearly every other child I knew, I was a bit afraid of the adults in my life – I always did what I was told, never answered back and was expected to keep all the other kids out of trouble. I idolised my parents, my teachers and my aunts and uncles. The idea of ever displeasing or disappointing them was unthinkable. The few times I had were burned in my memory as shameful experiences of rejection which from then on I tried to avoid at all costs.

Television was rationed – the only times I remember being allowed to watch it for hours on end were during school holidays. It certainly wasn't on at meal times. My parents were foodies and great cooks, and everything they dished up was delicious. With four kids to feed, meals had to be kept simple – lots of hearty stews, roast vegetables and joints of meat, sausages and mash, and my mum's lamb's fry, which we all loved, especially the rich oniony gravy the slightly chewy meat came in. In the summer, virtually every night involved a barbecue of some kind. If you wanted seconds, it was first come, first served, so I developed a lightning-fast eating technique so I could enjoy as much as possible. Moderation wasn't in my vocabulary.

The only meal I hated was breakfast, because I was never hungry first thing in the morning and found Weet-Bix and toast about as exciting as a doctor's waiting room. At other times of the day, my appetite knew no bounds. I dreamed of inhabiting a world like the one in the Enid Blyton books I devoured, where there were magical forests with chocolate trees, ice-cream mountains, toffee flowers and rain that tasted of sherbet. Food was delicious, comforting and also very interesting. My mother and both my grandmothers taught me how to cook, which I loved. I could make Anzac biscuits or pancakes quite confidently on my own by the age of nine. I even once made homemade pasta, but couldn't roll it thinly enough because we didn't have a pasta machine, so the meal ended up being lumps of dough. (My family lovingly ate it anyway, bless them.)

But everything changed once I started my last year of primary school. All of a sudden, I shot up to my full adult height (175 centimetres) and started filling out, which we were told at school was normal for girls. But normal was the last thing I felt. The physical changes in me brought about a whole heap of problems because, although I would have violently protested to the contrary, I was not mature for my age.

When you're sixteen or seventeen, getting hit on by pervy blokes at barbecues might be a bit of an ego boost. But when you're barely twelve, you still have Cabbage Patch dolls on your bed, and the most romantic movie you've ever watched is *The Sound of Music*, it's pretty bloody terrifying.

I began to feel betrayed by my body. It was something other people were noticing now, whereas before I'd just been this annoying little kid who could scamper about naked under the sprinklers without a care in the world and didn't have the faintest clue what all her various bits were for. I was still that child, but now in an adult's body.

Food, all of a sudden, became a huge issue. I'd always had a big appetite for both food and books – when I ran out of Enid Blytons or Baby-Sitters Clubs, I used to fall on the pile of women's magazines my mum and nan (who lived a few streets away) liked to read. I began to notice that all of them had recipes for delicious-looking food, but they also had sections full of the latest diets: the Israeli Army diet, which involved eating only apples for two days, then only cheese for two days, then chicken, and so on until you were bored into a coma; and the Superwoman diet, which mostly consisted of grapefruit, dry biscuits and packet soup – foods I didn't associate with being a powerful woman. But oh boy, did these aspirational articles work on a naive little mind like mine. I remember thinking, 'If only I was a grown-up and had my own house and actually got to decide what I ate. Then I'd be thin.'

Around this time, an old family friend came to visit. After greeting her, we kids left the adults to it. As I walked away, she said to me, 'Wow, Philippa! You're a *big* girl.'

She didn't mean tall. I'd read enough women's magazines to know what she meant.

I'd love to tell you that I was a feisty almost-teenager and my sense of justice was so finely honed that I asked her, 'Where do you get off, saying that to a sweet, impressionable, normal-looking kid? Don't you realise you're perpetuating the cycle of women only feeling they are worthwhile and attractive if they're thin? Why does what I look like matter so much? Doesn't it matter that I get good grades at school? That I'm a good sister and a good friend? And that one day I'll write a book that will change the world?' (Dear reader, you are, of course, holding that book.)

But of course, that didn't happen. Not only would I have been in deep trouble for talking back to a grown-up – a guest, no less – it didn't even occur to me that she was wrong. If an adult had said it, it must be true. I was *big*. Many years later I found a picture of all of us taken that day. Admittedly I didn't look skinny and I certainly didn't look as young as I was – I could have been plonked in a bar and only the most diligent of the staff would have asked me for ID. But as far as size was concerned, I wasn't *big*.

From that moment on, every casual remark or commentary about my size, appearance or appetite got tucked away into my *I am fat, I am disgusting* file. Food was no longer something I allowed myself to take any pleasure in. I ripped all the latest diet plans out of the magazines and kept them in my bedside table so I could memorise the foods I was allowed and the foods I wasn't. Fat was now the enemy. I ate a lot of dry chicken burgers from the school tuckshop, always asking for no mayonnaise. Baked potatoes and crispbreads were also eaten dry. I put no cheese on my pasta. If I saw oil being used in the preparation of a dish I knew I would have to eat, I had a panic attack. This was also the era when the super-model was the new celebrity, so every time I opened a magazine there was yet another perfect body to measure my own against, to push my self-esteem a little lower.

I had now started high school and we all know what a kind, comforting place that is for an insecure kid who's a bit 'unique', as most of my teachers described me in my reports. And an all-girls school, of course, is even more of a haven for the slightly socially inept and naive. Being bullied became a part of my daily routine, like brushing my teeth. Writing this now, over twenty years later, I struggle to recall the exact details because I've had hypnotherapy to banish these memories. They are wrapped in chains, padlocked and behind a tree somewhere now ... at least, that's what my hyp-notherapist told me to do with them. But I remember there being some kind of sexual propositioning by much older girls that left me feeling dirty and frightened. My friends did nothing because they were also terrified of these older, bigger girls. I confessed as much as I could bear to my diary, feeling sick just writing the words. My parents eventually discovered the diary and hence the bullying. They were furious – inadvertently making my shame and guilt worse, because I thought if my parents were angry about something that involved me, it must have been my fault – and went to the school. I had already warned Mum and Dad what the principal's reaction would be. The one time I had complained about bullying to her, she'd said, 'What would Jesus do?'

I will freely admit that I have a sensitive nature, so the normal ups and downs of adolescence were probably harder because of that. But life, especially at school, was often traumatic and confusing, so I retreated almost permanently into a fantasy world. My increasing size wasn't helped by the fact I'd stopped playing sport once I started high school. Thanks to the recession Australia had to have, my family had sold up our house in the city and moved to a cheaper area in the countryside, about 60 kilometres away from school, which meant sports practice, school socials and drama productions were now out. Writing, something I had always loved doing, therefore became my new refuge. I wrote novels, stories, poems, scripts and songs, pouring everything out. Now that my teenage years were in full swing, it was the only thing that kept me sane.

That, and the chocolate cream biscuits that were always in the cupboard. My parents have a tendency to grocery shop as if an apocalypse is about to happen, so there was always about a month's supply of biscuits in the pantry. I would get through at least one packet of them on my own every day after school. As I tapped away on the typewriter (mid-1990s, remember), conjuring up worlds I longed to live in instead of one where I had no power and no respect, one filled with exams, bullies on the bus, and boys I liked but who made it clear they didn't like me back, I'd eat the entire packet of biscuits, one by one, mechanically, barely pausing between the final swallow of the last biscuit and the first bite of the next. Every bite gave me a rush, a comfort, a sugar high, and I didn't want it to stop.

Every day I woke up and told myself I wasn't going to do this any more, that this would be the day everything would be okay again. Every evening, when the same old sadness, guilt and confusion had swamped me, I would sneak a packet of biscuits into my bedroom and open a book or put a piece of paper into my typewriter.

I binged like this not just for obvious reasons, but also because during the rest of the day, certainly when I was around other people, I ate as little as possible, sometimes nothing at all. People had commented on my large appetite a couple of times, which had made me very self-conscious about eating in front of others. I would get through the day having barely eaten and then fall on whatever I could find as soon as I got home from school. I had to do it while no one was looking, because getting caught eating between meals usually resulted in a 'Why are you eating? It's nearly dinner time, don't have so many! Leave some for everyone else! How can you possibly be hungry?' inquisition, which I tried to avoid as much as possible. I'd flagellate myself for my lack of self-control. In health class at school, we'd watch videos about girls with eating disorders and I'd think, 'Maybe I just need to stop eating. Then I'll be thin. Then the bullying will stop. Then boys will notice me. Then people will be nice to me.'

At this point my parents started to cotton on that all was not well in the world of Phil, but they were not trained psychologists, which is probably what the situation needed. Instead, they used the same technique they had used on me as a young child to snap me out of silly behaviour – fear. If I didn't sort myself out, there would be consequences. They were watching me. It was the emotional equivalent of the naughty corner. I was terrified of upsetting and disappointing them, but at the same time there was a black cloud in my head that I couldn't get rid of and that no one seemed to understand. So I had to start getting crafty about my starving and bingeing. If there was any food left in my lunchbox when I came home from school, unable to waste food by throwing it away, I would hide it in my wardrobe. But Mum eventually found the stash of muesli bars, rice cakes and dried fruits stuffed behind my piles of over-sized Sportsgirl T-shirts, and she hit the roof. There was no real explanation I could offer that would satisfy her, because the truth would cause even more trouble. Trying to articulate my needs, and telling people how I felt and what I wanted from them, was a bit like rollerskating with my eyes shut: impossible to do without falling on my face. In my experience, telling people the truth usually lead to hurting their feelings, which, in my desire to be good, I always wanted to avoid. But pretending everything was okay was not equipping me to make the best choices – something I would pay for later.

Meanwhile, I threw myself into my school work. I had some wonderful teachers and praise from them went some way to repairing my fragile sense of self-worth and fed my longing for acceptance. I was an attentive student and read constantly, filling my head with details of life in England during the First World War, the gods of Hinduism, film stars of the 1940s, the entire Kennedy family dynasty. I had an indefatigable thirst for knowledge about the world and its people. By the time I was fifteen, I had about the same number of penpals all over the world, from countries as diverse as the USA, Japan or Uzbekistan. My penpals in Germany even got letters from me in my basic German. I gulped down all my penpals' letters, marvelled over their fascinating lives – even though they were just going to school like I was – and longed to meet them in person.

My dad was something of a kindred spirit; we both loved music and spent many hours jamming in his music room or singing Beatles songs at the top of our lungs in the car when he drove me home from school. My mum and I would spend time together sewing or doing crafty projects, which I found to be great fun. I loved spending time with my sisters, particularly inventing games with bizarre characters and storylines to make them laugh. Nature was another outlet for me – I loved to walk along the beach or, once we moved back to the city, in the bushland near my home, or through Dad's neat rows of vegetables, picking snowpeas off the vine. Sitting among the jasmine, roses and lavender in my parents' garden was like aromatherapy come to life.

I avoided sport as much as possible, and P.E. was my most dreaded class, especially if it involved a public weigh-in. I remember a few girls moaning, 'Oh my God, I'm 63 kilos! I'm so fat!' and wanting to slap them. I hadn't been 63 kilograms since I was twelve. By this time I was fifteen and weighed 91 kilograms. Much to my frustration, all this starving and bingeing had not had the desired effect. When I was cast in the title role in the school's production of *Toad of Toad Hall*, my well-connected drama teacher managed to get the costumes used by the Hobart theatre company that had put on the same play the year before in the Botanical Gardens. The role of Toad had been played by a rather rotund gentleman and the costume he had worn was a perfect fit on me.

In January 1997, I had left my high school and would be starting Year 11 in a few weeks' time at one of Hobart's most prestigious private schools, where I had won a scholarship. I was several months away from turning sixteen. This was when we discovered that I no longer fitted into the expensive school uniform bought for me. Losing weight was not just pure vanity any more, it was of economic necessity! To everyone's surprise, I managed to get my trousers done up by the time school started, and by third term I had shed 20 kilograms by following a low-fat, low-calorie diet and regular exercise, which was a bit of a drag but I did it anyway, fuelled by embarrassment, if nothing else. But I loved my new school, where my talents were recognised and encouraged. The bullies I'd hated at my old school were gone. In the pre-Facebook world, once people were out of your daily life, you tended never to see or hear from them again. Not only did I have new friends, I had control over which subjects I studied, so I did nothing but drama, literature, languages and history and loved every second of it. People had also noticed my weight loss. I'd been a rather heavy girl when I'd started, but by the time the school formal rolled around in November, I was resplendent in a size 12 green and silver gown. Jaws visibly dropped when I walked into the Grand Chancellor ballroom. Having never had this kind of attention in my life, it was like a drug.

Studying for my HSC the following year was a whole new world of pressure. I crammed and crammed but it was difficult to get peace and quiet in a rowdy house like my family's. I began to panic that I just wasn't going to do as well as I, and my parents and teachers, hoped. The HSC was the be-all and end-all, it seemed, and with these rising feelings of inadequacy, combined with the fact the attention from my dramatic weight loss the year before was drying up, my newly minted self-esteem fractured under the pressure and I coped with these scary feelings the only way I knew how. But instead of starving and bingeing, this time I just starved.

Every day became a battle. Every meal time was a gauntlet to run. At breakfast I would conceal mouthfuls of cereal in my cheeks that I would spit out at the earliest opportunity, and then go to classes at school where I could barely concentrate. This went on for the best part of two months and eventually my favourite teacher realised what was happening and phoned my parents. The guilt I felt at worrying my family slowly snapped me out of this behaviour, but I didn't see their concern as love. I saw it as, 'You are a bad person for making us worry.' Where did all this self-hate come from? I wasn't a bad kid. My family loved me. I had friends. Why did I think I was basically Hitler trapped in an Australian teenager's body? I had no compassion for myself at all. My sense of self was so fragile and I believed there was something profoundly disappointing about me.

My HSC results arrived and I had achieved a perfect score – 100 out of 100. The University of Tasmania offered me a scholarship. I had so many dreams and plans of all the marvellous things I was going to do and see and write and achieve. I watched my classmates leave Hobart in droves to accept places at universities on the mainland or take gap years climbing mountains in Peru or working at boarding schools in the UK. Why wasn't I going with them?

This is where I want to shake seventeen-year-old Phil.

Well, actually, what I want to do is sit her down with a cup of chamomile tea and calmly explain to her *all the shit that will go down* if she stays.

But I know why she stayed. She loved her family and couldn't imagine life without them. She adored her younger sisters and didn't want to miss out on anything in their lives. Growing up in a small town does one of two things to a person – it either breeds a fierce desire for independence and adventure, so you leave as soon as you can or it gives you Hotel California syndrome (as in, you can check out whenever you want but . . .) In my heart I was the former but told myself I was the latter. I wanted so badly to belong there. The idea of having to face the big wide world alone was terrifying. I was so passive, always waiting for permission, for validation or acceptance – even my wildest dreams of being an actor or a writer were fenced in by my presumption that I could only do either if I was 'discovered' first. And yet, underneath, there was a fire, a burning, an insatiable curiosity about the world, a fierce longing to break free, to see and do and feel and know. I was desperate to escape from everything I'd ever known, and yet the fear became stronger than the fire.

I still had one final detour to make before I started finding my way out.

Down the aisle.

An enclosed basin

'Having embarked on your marital voyage,
it is impossible not to be aware that you make
no way and that the sea is not within sight –
that, in fact, you are exploring an enclosed basin.'

– GEORGE ELIOT, *MIDDLEMARCH*

As tempting as it is to paint my teenage self as a hopeless romantic, the reality is I was just hopeless. Like most girls my age, I was obsessed with boys, kissing and losing my virginity, and terrified of all those things at the same time. To find myself blowing out candles on my eighteenth birthday cake with no boyfriend on the horizon was beyond embarrassing. My younger sisters were being asked out on dates, even having red roses left for them in the letterbox. The closest I had ever had to any of that was a bizarre, romantic-looking card from my penpal in Uzbekistan a few years earlier, an indecipherable Russian phrase on the front and passionate declarations written on the inside, suggesting he come to Australia to meet me. I was secretly relieved when Vladik stopped writing to me, but also deflated because there was nothing else on offer. I had hoped to meet someone at university but was disappointed to discover that the only guys in my classes to take a shine to me were ones with behavioural ticks or severe body odour issues.

I didn't get it. I told boys I liked them, then ignored them. The one time I had gone to a nightclub – Regine's, a staple in Hobart's skeletal night scene at the time – some random guy had tried to kiss me on the dance floor, cheap vodka potent on his breath, and I freaked out and ran away. I dressed like an Amish woman, my favourite outfit being an ankle-length black skirt from Target coupled with a denim blouse typical of the fashion at the time. Form an orderly queue, young men of 1999!

Despite no longer being in the grips of the eating disorder that had plagued my last year at school, I was still paranoid about my appearance because I had put on weight once I started eating (somewhat) normally again and was back in size 14 clothes. I didn't exercise. I spent my days studying, reading, working at my casual job on the weekends, driving around in my car (which I affectionately named 'The Beast'), and trying to write the Great Australian Novel. I was filled mostly with Diet Coke, jelly babies and a handful of cigarettes I'd dared to smoke before my father caught me one day, but I was also filled with longing. Longing to escape. Longing to be taken seriously. Longing for attention, adoration, love. There was a restlessness inside me I couldn't name.

*

'Why the hell would I go to ballroom dancing classes?' I asked Mum when she brought up the idea.

'I think it would be good for you,' she said, folding the laundry. My job was to sort the socks and I sat there with her stiffly as I rolled them into neat pairs. 'You're young, you should be getting out and meeting people.'

In other words, 'Why haven't you got a boyfriend yet?' I was self-conscious enough already about that fact; the idea that other people had noticed the opposite sex's lack of interest in me was deeply embarrassing.

'I can't go on my own,' I moaned.

But Mum had already pre-empted that excuse and recruited my younger sister Claire, nearly fifteen at the time, to join me at beginner's lessons on Wednesday nights. There was no way out, it seemed.

'Come on, you love *Strictly Ballroom*!' Mum tried to psych me up.

What was the subtext? I wondered sulkily. Was I Fran, the spotty, awkward girl with two left feet? If I just fixed my hair, put on a decent dress and took off those glasses, would my Scott be waiting there in the studio for me?

On Wednesday night, Claire and I were there at the dance studio but Paul Mercurio was nowhere to be seen. We started learning the box step, the foxtrot, the salsa, the waltz. It was actually quite fun and once I let go of the expectation I'd be undergoing a transformation worthy of a Baz Luhrmann film and got the hang of the steps, I started to feel remarkably graceful. I began to look forward to Wednesday nights. Dancing was great exercise and I was delighted to find my clothes were looser as a result. As we became more confident dancers, Claire and I started staying for the social dance after the lessons. My favourite was the rumba, and to my great surprise, I was asked to dance quite a lot by the men who attended the socials.

At some point over the weeks that followed, during a class I was introduced to a guy a few years older than me, with blue eyes, sandy brown hair and a kind face. His name was Glenn. As women outnumbered men significantly in the beginners class and he was an experienced dancer, he'd been roped in as an extra partner by the teachers. I don't remember meeting him for the first time, or how we got talking. Most likely he told me one of the jokes in his repertoire and I laughed, possibly the first woman alive to do so.

Things continued in this way each Wednesday night for a month or so – we would smile and chat briefly whenever we were partnered together as the beginners made their way around the circle – and then I found myself bumping into him at university on other days as well. Glenn was twenty-one to my eighteen, and he was in the fourth year of his degree. Initially I'd thought this was because he was doing an honours year, but in fact it was because he hadn't yet passed enough subjects to graduate! In those early days we never really hung out and talked properly; we just had fleeting conversations as we passed each other on campus. I found myself looking forward to running into him and whenever I did, I got all nervous and flustered. I hadn't felt this way about anyone before, apart from Kieren Perkins and Brian from the Backstreet Boys. It got to the stage where I thought about Glenn nearly all the time. But what made this exciting was the possibility that something would actually happen – the Backstreet Boys were hardly hanging around in the Elizabeth Street mall, so I could forget about Brian. This was a flesh and blood man in front of me, and he seemed to like me too.

Glenn was a great dancer and his confidence was infectious. We swept across the dance floor together very comfortably and not once did I trip over my size 11 feet (and nor did he). We danced every dance that I knew and then we would sit on the side and talk, occasionally interrupted by older ladies who wanted to snatch him away for a more complex step I didn't know, and as the weeks went by, we sat closer and closer. He nearly always wore a leather jacket – his twenty-first birthday present, he told me – which smelled like the seats in the car I'd learned to drive in. It was familiar and strangely comforting.

We also started emailing, mostly telling each other jokes. Some of his emails, looking back, were in quite poor taste (and in all honesty I didn't fully understand some of them). If I had a daughter I'd tell her to run a mile if a prospective boyfriend ever sent her jokes like that, but mostly they were just silly and typical of a bloke in his early twenties trying to big-note himself. I didn't really know much about anything. All I knew was that a man was showing an interest in me, and I liked it.

The thing about falling in love is that you don't decide to do it – it just happens. Falling out of love is the same. Neither Glenn nor I had any idea what we were getting into. We were both lonely, inexperienced and longing to be loved, but we were very different people. Born into a military family, Glenn had lived in nearly every state and territory of Australia, whereas I had never lived anywhere but Hobart. His pleasures were simple and his life revolved around sport – cricket in the summer; rugby, soccer and AFL in the winter. He was a smart guy and had a very mathematical mind, but wasn't particularly studious or much of a reader. He didn't even have a library card, something I'd had since 1985. But the wide gaps in our interests didn't concern me at the time, nor did Glenn's social skills, which had been somewhat stunted thanks to moving around so much during his childhood. Making friends wasn't his strongest talent. He wasn't shy but he was very competitive, which often made things awkward. Glenn had to be the best, at everything. He had to win, at everything. He was rarely gracious in defeat, whether it was a game of gin rummy or backyard cricket, so as you might expect, he was not the most popular guy on the planet.

Glenn's family was also very different to mine; in fact they were almost the very opposite, something I didn't realise straight away. One afternoon early in the relationship I was alone in their house. Glenn, his parents and siblings were all either at work or cricket until late. Their house was not the tidiest, certainly not compared to my family's, which was rarely anything less than pristine, even with four teenagers living in it. In my house there was always something that needed doing, so if you were home, you were expected to do it. I assumed Glenn's family was the same and that they'd be angry if I sat around watching TV all afternoon. So I cleaned the house for them. Within a few hours, the piles of newspapers were in the recycling, the week's worth of washing up was done, the years of dust were vacuumed up and polished away, and the air was fresh. I hoped my efforts would impress them. When they finally returned home, I didn't even get a chance to say hello before Glenn shot an amused look at his mother and said, 'I told you she'd clean the place, didn't I?'

His mother wasn't smiling. 'Have you been cleaning *my* house, Philippa?' she asked.

That was it. The black mark I got against me that day was never erased, a sharp contrast to how warmly my own family welcomed

Glenn into the fold. But instead of being concerned about this, I simply tried not to think about it, especially the fact that Glenn hadn't stood up for me.

Despite that, with each of us as inexperienced as the other, the first six months we were together were possibly the happiest time either of us had ever known. We went to the movies and held hands in the dark; we went on drives to Richmond, Huonville and New Norfolk and had picnics; and of course there were heated, bra-tangling moments whenever we found ourselves alone in either of our parents' houses. This was the first proper relationship of my life and I was euphoric. My anxieties about not being worthy of love were gone. I couldn't see that we were two very different people, and loneliness was all we really had in common. We came to each other empty, filling each other's lives like you would fill a bucket with water, failing to notice there was a hole in the bottom.

*

I remember being blindly enthusiastic about planning a life with Glenn. He bought me a small, inexpensive dress ring as a gift within a few months of us dating, and this made me wildly happy. I day-dreamed about our future, where we might live, the house we might have. I remember being very excited at the prospect of getting engaged, but the exact details of how that happened are now so murky. Did I pressure him? Or did he want freedom and independence as badly as I did? We were officially engaged by the spring of 2000, only a year after we'd first met, and while our families and friends were congratulatory and supportive, there was an undercurrent of concern. I was only nineteen. My parents said that all they cared about was that I was happy. The looks in their eyes were not of pride, I remember now, but of caution. 'Why don't you just live together first?' they gently suggested.

Looking back, I can see I was rebelling, as silly as that sounds. I might have been young and immature, but I was now legally an adult. I didn't have to do what my parents told me or thought was best. I wanted to be a grown-up. I wanted freedom. Yet, on the other hand, I didn't have the confidence to strike out on my own and was blissfully naive about the ways of the world. I only saw what I wanted to see. I wish I had known better but I simply didn't. My enthusiasm for settling down so young was foolish, to put it kindly. Anyone who tried to tell me that was rewarded with a wall of indifference. But despite their concerns, my parents were nothing but supportive. They knew trying to stop me would only end in tears.

By devoting myself to Glenn as quickly and completely as I did, I also missed out on an important part of university life: socialising and meeting different people. I fancied myself as too grown up for these activities and I didn't have time for anything non-academic. I spent every waking moment either with Glenn, at my lectures or tutorials, doing assignments or at my casual job, earning money that I never allowed myself to spend. Even when a script I wrote won the university's annual one-act play competition, I couldn't be unglued from Glenn's side. The play was performed on the Hobart campus and then toured Tasmania as part of the Deloraine Drama Festival. I didn't attend any rehearsals or get to know any of the cast or crew, despite being invited to do so. I just went along to the performance, where I sat in the audience, thrilled that actors were performing lines I had written. Glenn sat next to me in the theatre, squeezing my hand proudly, and that was all I cared about. You would have thought this early taste of success with my writing would have spurred me on. Instead, that was the last thing I wrote for some time. I was preparing for my next role – bride-to-be.

*

The year leading up to our wedding wasn't the easiest for either of us, with Glenn unable to find work after he graduated, but I think we both felt too invested in the relationship by then and were afraid to address the idea that we weren't as compatible as we had belie-ved. And I was too insecure to confront Glenn about things that bothered me. I told myself, and others who were concerned, that once we were married, things would be different.

And so we were married, from a place of hope and love, excited by the potential we had and what the future might hold, but oblivi-ous to what marriage actually entailed. We were happy at first, I think, but in devoting myself entirely to him I gave away everything, including my still-developing identity. It was 2002, but the way I was acting it might as well have been the 1950s. Compromise wasn't in Glenn's vocabulary and it was all I knew, so that was how our relationship worked. It wasn't perfect but by then, with my other dreams for the future shelved, it was all I had. I was now a wife, and that was about it. I had wanted it so badly but now I was there, it was clear I hadn't understood what it really meant at all.

Nevertheless, there were some lovely tender moments that first year – in fact, there had always been enough of them to silence the doubting voices in my head. A month after our wedding we were broke, but Glenn still managed to find the money to buy me some earrings I loved as a Valentine's Day present. He hid them in our new flat and wrote little poems as clues for me to find and follow, like a treasure hunt. One of them was hidden in the breadmaker, the clue being, 'You and I are newlywed, but not as new as fresh baked bread.' It was incredibly thoughtful and romantic, and unexpected, and my heart melted. Moments like that reassured me that I had made the right choice.

The year after we were married, 2003, was a dark year for me. I had just graduated from university, with first-class honours in English, and had planned to go on to postgraduate studies. However, the only way I could afford to do that was with a scholarship of some kind. For the first time in my life, I wasn't successful in obtaining one. As a result, I felt lost and hopeless. Looking back, I'm not sure what I was expecting – to walk out of my graduation ceremony, gowned and capped, and follow a sign clearly marked, 'Philippa, your destiny, this way'? I had been an overachieving student my entire life, a people-pleaser born and raised, with very few boundaries or life skills. I had been sheltered from a great deal. I had doggedly pursued my education and found, for all my lofty dreams and desires, that the real world was not all that thrilled I was there, out in the thick of it. But instead of realising that making your mark on the world requires courage, risk and that most precious of all commodities, time, I folded. I chose the most conventional path possible.

I was a deeply insecure young woman who refused to take responsibility for her own needs and expected those closest to her to be mind-readers. When I didn't get my needs met by others (and why would I, when I hadn't expressed them?), I sank further into self-pity, convinced this was further evidence of my unlovability. I had no idea how to assert myself or how to manage my emotions and keep my less helpful thoughts and behaviours in check. I let Glenn be in charge of nearly everything. He managed all the household finances and I lived on an allowance, even though I earned slightly more money than he did. Even though I had helped him learn to drive, whenever we went out somewhere together I would automatically walk to the passenger side of the car. In my school drama productions I had been used to playing the lead, but here I was, with a supporting role in my own life.

I gained a lot of weight, going from a size 12–14 to a size 20 in just one year. I stopped writing, even in a journal. Having been such a lover of words my whole life, being without them did something to my spirit and numbed me from the inside. I didn't even read any more, apart from cookbooks and glossy magazines filled with pictures of clothes I couldn't fit into or afford to buy, and exotic destinations that were so far out of my reach they might as well have been the moon.

My life at that time did not have the real me living in it, so it's really no wonder that I constantly felt misunderstood, unseen and unheard. I didn't even know who the real me was.

Things weren't helped by the fact that no one seemed to believe me when I tried to tell them how unhappy I was. To the outside world, everything probably looked fine and I was just 'being a drama queen', as always. I swallowed everything I was feeling, both literally and symbolically, because I was so afraid of rocking the boat. It felt self-indulgent to leave a reasonably well-paid job simply because I was miserable and wanted to do something else. It felt unreasonable to expect more from my relationship when my husband seemed quite content. This life I was living was the result of choices I had made freely. I had been a willing participant in everything. I had made my bed.

Life is short, the saying goes, unless you're miserable. Those two years, 2003 and 2004, were the longest of my life. My size 18 jeans got tighter, I now had full-blown adult acne and my typical afternoon tea was an entire cake. My job was stressful and boring. The brand-new home Glenn and I had lived in for barely six months felt like a tomb – the mortgage was exorbitant so quitting my job wasn't an option anyway. Instead of the happiness I'd anticipated in being married and having a house of my own, I just felt empty. The only thing I was excited about was finding my favourite Dove white chocolate priced to clear in Kmart for 67 cents a block. (I bought every single one.)

I was twenty-three, and I felt like my life was as good as over.

After one too many nights of binge-eating, with the tower of Dove now down to a few measly blocks, I finally worked up the courage to come clean to Glenn. I told him how unhappy I was in my job and that I'd reached the point where I didn't think I could keep going because I was worried about what I might do if I did. I was tired of feeling so worthless and sad all the time. What had happened to the ambitious girl, full of dreams, I used to be?

'I love us, but I hate me,' I sobbed.

Glenn had never been big on change, but he was surprisingly supportive. He agreed to sell the house so that I could quit my job and have some time out to think about what I really wanted to do with my life.

I pass that house, which we built together, every time I go home to Hobart. It looks okay, even pretty good, from the outside, but if you went inside, it would be clear it had been designed by a couple who didn't really know what they wanted and had no idea what they were doing.

With Glenn's support, I took a part-time job and once our house was sold we found a smaller, cheaper home to rent on the outskirts of West Moonah, with a lovely view over the Derwent River. Despite there being carpet in the kitchen and bathroom, it was cosy and seemed like the perfect place to start our next chapter, whatever that ended up being. Leaving my job had been the first step, but it certainly didn't solve all my problems because, of course, the job hadn't really been the problem at all. I spent the first few months of 2005 feeling out of my depth, and the chocolate binges continued in earnest. Denial was still my constant companion and I continued to tread water.

A month or so into my new job, I got an email from the editor of my old school's alumni magazine. She said she was doing a 'where are they now?' feature on 'all our top students' and wondered if I'd send her a few paragraphs about what I was up to. I sat at my desk and cried when I got that email. What on earth was I going to say? That I'd spent the seven years since I left school floundering around with little to show for myself? That I longed to travel but the furthest I'd ever ventured from Hobart was the Sunshine Coast? That despite losing 20 kilograms in Year 11, I had now put all that on again, plus more? That I was married to someone I loved very much, but who I was afraid deep down didn't really want the same things as me – and therefore I'd probably never get to do them?

The email went unanswered, as did every other wake-up call in early 2005. Until that day I sat with the donuts and recently developed photos in the shopping centre car park.

The scales don't lie

A few weeks after Anne joined Weight Watchers, she came around with a present for me – a Weight Watchers points guide. It was bright pink and wholesome-looking. 'Oh wow, Annie, that's lovely of you,' I leafed through the pages gingerly. 'How's it all going?'

'Great. I've lost 4 kilos already,' grinned Anne. 'It's pretty slow progress, but I'm feeling really good about it. The crew are pretty cool with it too. In fact, I don't think most of them have noticed.'

Anne lived in a share house filled with nineteen- and twenty-year-olds, who she referred to as 'the crew', in Launceston. At only twenty-three, she felt ten years older than them most of the time. Trying to eat healthily on a student's budget was proving to be a challenge, but she was managing. Ironically, she'd been able to buy tonnes of junk for her measly thirty-dollar weekly food budget.

I broke the news to Anne that I had decided I would follow the program with her because she had inspired me to start sorting myself out. Her face burst into a smile as she hugged me. 'But I can't afford to go to meetings so I'll weigh myself at home and text you with my results,' I said. 'That way we can keep each other motivated!'

So, after years of avoiding them, it was time for me to actually get on the scales. I could explain away mirror reflections, unflattering photos and clothing sizes but I couldn't deny whatever number the dial settled on. I would finally have numerical proof of how messy and out of focus my life had become.

I went into the bathroom and stripped down. Anne waited outside the door. I half expected to hear 'Eye of the Tiger' or some kind of ceremonial entering-the-ring music as I stepped on the scales. But I honestly had no idea how much my life was about to change in the next few seconds.

The dial of the scale swung violently, passing 100 kilograms. My heart sank as it finally settled on 103.5 kilograms. I felt sick with embarrassment as I put my clothes back on and came out, where Anne was waiting. I told her the number and let her put her arms around me as I cried.

According to the BMI charts, I was nearly 30 kilograms overweight. We sat down together and worked out that the maximum healthy weight for my height was 76 kilograms. The *maximum*. I had to lose nearly 28 kilograms to get to that point, just to not be classified as 'overweight' any more. How long was that going to take? It was hopeless. How had I let this happen?

'Well, my leader always says to those who have a lot to lose, just focus on the first 5 kilograms. Then you'll be feeling better and more confident about it all.' Anne put her head on my shoulder. 'I know you can do it. Thank you for doing this with me.'

I felt incredibly overwhelmed. It was all very well to see your problems in the harsh light of day, but where did you go from there? Was I strong enough to start changing things?

Somehow I knew I had to be.

Even now I'm still not sure what it was, but in that moment, on 25 April 2005, something in me snapped. The only way I can describe it is that I had a split-second but crystal-clear vision into what my future would be like if nothing changed. Suddenly, the sadness, self-pity and frustration at being so far from where I wanted to be just vanished. I needed a plan. I needed to be positive. I was not going to spend another minute of my life dissatisfied, broken-hearted, bored, negative, frightened and in a corner. All of that had to change and the only way it would was if I started, that very second, and didn't stop.

Normally, seeing 103.5 kilograms on the scale would have sent me into a spiral of depression and my emotional GPS would have directed me to the freezer for a 4-litre tub of ice-cream. But this time it was different. It wasn't a moment to feel depressed. It was a moment to celebrate. I was going to do something about it.

*

I had thrown myself into countless weight-loss schemes over the years so Glenn, unsurprisingly, thought this was just another false start. But over the weeks that followed I showed no signs of throwing in the towel. I think he was surprised to see me sticking to my plan. I'm sure he was hoping we would go back to eating KFC at least once a week, sometimes twice, having pizza and garlic bread every Friday night and watching football on the weekends with our usual orgy of chips and chocolate. He didn't seem all that happy that garlic bread had been dropped from pizza night and that the pizza itself was no longer thick and doughy but had thin, point-friendly pita breads as bases. And the cheese? It was now weighed in 30 gram increments. Every 30 grams was two Weight Watchers points and I had to watch every one of the twenty-two I was allowed each day. No, Glenn didn't like this. He didn't like it at all.

Even though I had Anne's support, I was going to need my husband's as well. My resolve was strong, but I needed all temptation out of the way. Our house would be a junk-free zone from now on, and he would have to eat whatever I did. Glenn had also put on a lot of weight since we got married and I felt this was something he needed to do too. At first, he was very resistant and told me to stop nagging. It didn't matter what I said; he wasn't interested. The change came a month or so into the program, when I emailed him the 'Weight Watchers for Men Gut Test'. I think Glenn thought that if he did this test it would shut me up for good, but it turned out he was well and truly in the 'danger zone', meaning that the weight he'd put on around his stomach was putting pressure on the vital organs in that part of the body. He reluctantly agreed then to try this plan with me. For a guy who rarely admitted any personal shortfalls, it was a real breakthrough. He might not have realised it, but I was truly grateful for his support. I had grown so used to us having very separate interests, so doing something together for a change was quite wonderful. All of a sudden there seemed to be some real closeness between us. I hadn't felt that way for a while.

One crucial thing I realised during this time was that all my other attempts at losing weight and getting my fitness under control had been fuelled by my shame and hatred of my overweight body, which I'd seen as a personal failure. This time my mindset had noticeably shifted. I wasn't tracking Weight Watchers points and going for a power walk every night because I hated myself; these were actually the first acts of self-love I had committed in my nearly twenty-four years on the planet. I wanted to get fit and healthy more than I could ever remember wanting anything in my life, and therefore I was prepared to put in the effort of healthy eating and exercise. I had some goals and I was actually going to try to reach them, instead of wandering through my life in a daze, full of food that never satisfied, with a body that ached from lack of movement and a soul that was deprived of any real nourishment. Reading travel books with my morning coffee no longer felt like I was indulging in pipe dreams. With every kilo I shed, I was ironically starting to think a bit bigger.

My diligence started to pay off. In two short months I was down by nearly 10 kilograms (as was Glenn) and for the first time in my life, I felt genuinely proud of myself. I was actually sticking to something! My clothes fit better, and although most people were yet to comment on any difference in my appearance, I felt happier and more confident than I'd felt in years. Life suddenly seemed to have a bit more purpose. Instead of watching TV all the time, Glenn and I started exercising together and took any opportunity to be active. After work and on weekends we would power walk together around the streets, climbing the various inclines of West Moonah to the fringe of Lenah Valley until we were red-faced, sweaty and puffing.

My thighs ached after these power walks. I wondered if I would ever be fit enough to run. It seemed impossible.

We were both enjoying our new healthy meals too. Our former dinners of mountains of pasta, potatoes and rice were out – our plates were now piled high with lean grilled meat, salad, chargrilled zucchini and capsicum and steamed corn cobs. Any carbs we had were measured carefully. I'd had no idea what a healthy portion of pasta or rice really looked like – what I had always thought of as two cups was actually more of a Pavarotti-sized portion. Kitchen scales and measuring cups were indispensable while I was learning. Gone were the giant tubs of cheap ice-cream which the two of us usually got through in a weekend. Now we bought individually portioned cups of low-fat ice-cream which, to our great surprise, were rather tasty. It was unexpectedly gratifying to be exercising such restraint, to be savouring these smaller portions and once-a-week treats, to go to bed feeling light and looking forward to breakfast – to look forward to every meal, come to think of it.

I had started tracking all my food, points and weigh-in results in a notebook and had also decided to use it as an anchor in case my resolve ever wavered. I dug out the photos that had made me recoil in horror in the car at Kmart that day a few months ago, when I'd crammed cinnamon donuts into my mouth as a method of stifling my fear and disgust at what I'd seen and what I knew I had become. I pasted those photos into the notebook. I took a huge black marker and wrote underneath them, 'I don't want this to be me.' My tracker became a diary of sorts, recording my days, triumphs, new starts. Every time I was tempted to chuck it all in, every time

I wanted to have a donut-cramming session, every time I was tempted to eat to stifle any negative feelings, I would get out this notebook, turn to these photos and allow my desire for change to overwhelm the urge to eat. Becoming conscious of what I had actually been doing to myself had frightened me. A bright torch had been shone on my behaviour, my clumsy and uncaring ways of dealing with my problems. But instead of running away, I was facing it.

Having embraced healthy living with gusto, I was also noticing 'non-scale victories'. These can be any way to measure your progress other than the scales, such as being able to run up a hill rather than walk, your blood pressure dropping, your clothes being looser, your wedding rings not being as tight. For me, it was shoes.

It's hard to feel sexy and feminine when you have to buy your shoes from the chemist. I had longed for a pair of gorgeous winter boots and had tried, and failed, to buy some many times over the years. My calves were so wide and meaty that trying on boots was like trying to put a football into a wine bottle. The zips rarely made it past my ankles. But, buoyed by the general looseness of my skirts and trousers, I found myself wandering into the Moonah Harris Scarfe department store on my way home from work. There were mid-calf boots on sale and I found some in a size 11. They were tight, but they did up, all the way. Letting this miraculous news sink in, I sat down quietly on the chair near the mirror and stared at my feet and calves in these sleek, black boots, which seemed to have transformed my clown feet into something elegant. I was bursting with pride.

I got the boots! I texted Anne after lugging the precious cargo back to the car.

Anne texted back immediately. *Fab news babe! Did I tell you I'm going to Thailand in September? You should totally come!! You'll be in a bikini by then* ☺

I hesitated before pressing send on my reply. *We'll probably be living in Melbourne by then.*

Melbourne or bust

I didn't keep a journal during 2003 and 2004, so I don't really remember how or when Glenn and I started to think about moving interstate to Melbourne. When I started journalling again properly in June 2005, the move was already fully on the table but I was writing about it with a curious mixture of excitement and trepidation. 'I told myself I didn't want to keep a diary until I felt excited by life again,' I wrote on the first creamy page of the silk-covered notebook I'd bought in a beautiful shop in Noosa on my honeymoon three years earlier but never written in. Now both Glenn and I were excited about the future for the first time in years. It was a happy time for us. Being on the edges of our comfort zone as a couple was exhilarating, certainly in comparison with the years we'd spent together so far. A part of me was very frightened of what leaving Tasmania would mean – fear had certainly made me put it off long enough – but an even bigger part of me had started to hope in earnest.

Glenn got a transfer with the company he worked for and now the plans for our new life in Melbourne could really start. I resigned from my job; we booked movers and a passage on the *Spirit of Tasmania*. I had also applied to the University of Melbourne to start postgraduate study the following year. Everything was falling into place. I was heartened by how keen Glenn was on this change too, how ready he was for an adventure, something new. It all felt very exciting.

It wasn't easy to leave, however. I knew I would miss my family terribly. I had grown closer to them over the past few months. Taking control of my health and fitness had made me a bit more confident and I began to open up more to people. I actually shared things with them when I was feeling down rather than swallowing everything. I also started to feel my love of writing come back. That thick journal slowly began filling up and I had an uplifting conversation with a colleague at work, a talented and recently award-winning novelist, that really fired me up. 'The only thing to do with your dreams is to *do* them,' she said passionately. 'Fortune favours the bold. If this is what you want to do with your life, you have to go for it.'

But of course, the move to Melbourne meant having to leave this new job, where I had only been for about nine months. I was a bit sad about it, as it had been very satisfying and interesting work and I had enjoyed autonomy for the first time in my career. I had loved being able to manage my own time rather than being constantly watched, as I had been at my last job. My departure, while disappointing, was not unexpected – apparently I had mentioned in my interview that a move interstate was something I was thinking about in the near future (probably my answer to the dreaded 'where do you see yourself in five years?' question). But when I had a farewell cup of tea with one of my managers, who wanted to know my plans for my new life in Melbourne, her reaction caught me off guard.

'Oh, lord. Not another girl who wants to be a writer. There's no money in it. The writing world is so competitive. And that's if you're even any good.' She cast an eye over me, as if to say, *which you clearly aren't*. 'It's not for the weak-hearted, you know. Ninety-nine per cent of people shouldn't even bother trying.'

I was struck dumb by her bluntness. Barely pausing for breath, she fired her next question. 'What's your back-up plan?'

In a very small voice, I replied, 'Well, I was going to get a Dip. Ed. and teach high school English.'

'Oh no, you've got too much of a Pollyanna outlook on life to stick that out.'

Apparently, my manager thought that high-school teaching would be disastrous for me because I was such a gentle spirit (a pushover, in other words) and all the teenage shitheads I'd have to teach would inevitably crush me.

'You'd be better suited to primary school teaching,' she said definitely. 'Much better. Simpler life for you.'

Perhaps I should have argued with her, and perhaps she wanted me to, to show a bit of spark, a bit of fire. Instead, I just sat there, meek and stupefied, fulfilling her every perception of me. After the lovely conversation I'd had with my other colleague, who had been nothing but positive and encouraging, this was a real sting. I did my best to hide my devastation and ignore the voice in my head that said, 'Well, she knows what she's talking about. You must be no good, if she thinks so.' Looking back, I can of course see that she was right about a couple of things, especially writing not being for the weak-hearted. I probably needed a reality check so I didn't get too carried away. But at the time I was quite deflated.

A few months prior, I would have stopped at Banjo's Bakehouse on the way home for a few apple danishes to make me feel better. Instead, I went round to my parents' house to say hello and I told Mum and my youngest sister, Rebekah, what my manager had said to me.

'You'll prove her wrong, I know you will,' Mum said with conviction.

Rebekah went into the study and came out with a magazine. It was a publication her school had put out at the end of 2003, featuring the creative work of students in Years 9–12. She had been featured in it, and in the notes on the contributors there was this line in my sister's entry: 'Rebekah says her major source of inspiration for her writing is her older sister, Philippa.' She had never shown this to me before. Even Glenn, when I told him what had happened, comforted me and told me he believed in me.

I felt so chastened by their kindness. It was funny – now that I was feeling a bit more comfortable in my own skin, reaching out to people was so much easier. I began to realise I didn't have to do it all on my own. When I was upset, I didn't have to bottle it up, because no one cared. Quite the opposite. And as for a simpler life, well, that was the last thing in the world I wanted. I was under no illusions it would be easy but I was damned if I was going to give up when I'd only just started trying again.

Another reason I was looking forward to moving to Melbourne was because there would be, at least not straight away, no sporting club into which all of Glenn's free time would disappear. Not that Glenn wasn't entitled to pursue his own interests; it just felt like we never got much quality time together. Things I wanted to do, that I wanted to share with him, nearly always had to be put on the back-burner. I loved the idea that maybe we would have weekends to do fun, cool Melbourne-couple things like shop for organic vegetables at the Queen Victoria Market, stroll along Southbank or the St Kilda boardwalk, take in a show at the Malthouse and have lattes in Federation Square. Maybe we could finally have a summer holiday too.

The more I thought about it, the more I liked the idea of living somewhere else. I wanted to belong in Hobart so badly – mostly so that I wouldn't have to leave the people I loved – but I yearned deeply for something else. A release, a reinvention, a chance to create a life entirely on my own terms. I didn't have any firm idea what I would be doing in six months' time – apart from going back to university, as Glenn and I had discussed – but nothing was set in stone any more. This thrilled me. Finally, life was going to be exciting. I was no longer a victim of my own excuses or other people's expectations. With every day that passed, every kilogram that left my body, every blouse or skirt that was too loose now, every time I made a herbal tea instead of cutting a wedge of cake, we got closer to Melbourne and I felt the old life, the old me, slip further away.

What's a blog?

n 2005, the internet was like a kid learning to ride a bike. The
training wheels were still on and most of us had barely scratched
the surface of what truly lay out there on the web. I was a huge
fan of blogs in these early years and they were nothing like the mini
magazines they mostly are today. Back then, they were like diaries:
honest, not as polished. Most of the ones I followed were either
food blogs, full of interesting recipes and anecdotes about the writers' lives (which were way more exciting than mine), or the blogs
of writers I admired. Some writers were established and published;
others were just like me, wondering if anything would ever come
of the snatches of poetry they wrote during their lunchbreaks.

After making the decision to get my health and fitness under
control, I found myself regularly scrolling through the Weight

Watchers Australia website, scribbling down ideas and recipes to try, motivational nuggets that I could write in my tracker. One day I clicked on 'Members' blogs' and discovered the online journals of women all over the country who were following the plan. These were another weapon in my weight-loss motivational arsenal. I didn't have an internet connection at home so I went to work early each day so I had time to catch up with my virtual friends. There were two women based in Sydney I found particularly motivating – a young mum to two children, living on Sydney's north shore, who referred to herself by her first initial, M; and Mary, in her late twenties and living with her boyfriend in funky Newtown. I was unfamiliar with the areas they described but was entranced all the same. I read about M doing a daily lunchtime walk in the Domain, breathing in the bustling air of Sydney Harbour, and about Mary's adventures at boot camp in Hyde Park and going to yoga classes. I pictured them both, walking along the streets littered with frangipani flowers, drinking coffee in fancy cafes. But they certainly didn't glamourise their lives – they talked about their struggles, their relief when a bad day, week or month had passed but they had managed to stay on track, the buzz they got from exercise, their hopes for the future. I felt exactly the same! As the months went by I silently rejoiced with M and Mary as they continued to succeed, and realised there was a small but growing weight-loss community online. I found myself on other blogs written by women in New Zealand, the UK and America. Reading about how these ordinary women fit their exercise into a busy day, what they cooked for dinner and their growing sense of self-esteem was so motivating, and I eagerly lapped up the details. Every success story fired me up. I felt like I knew these people, and I grew to rely on them for daily company and support, even though I had never left a single comment.

It was in Melbourne, merely two weeks after getting off the boat, that I began to think about starting a blog of my own. I wasn't going to be getting a job straight away, as I was planning to start post-graduate study in a few months, so I was going to have to meet people some other way. I wanted to be a part of the online camaraderie I had come to admire so much, to join in the conversation. The past five months had made me feel proud of myself, like what I had achieved (13 kilograms down, 14.5 to go) was worth celebrating and talking about. I no longer wanted to hide under a rock. And who knew? Maybe I could help and inspire other people too, like the bloggers I read daily inspired me.

I was sipping a latte in the City Library cafe in Flinders Lane, doodling in a notebook and brainstorming potential blog names. I tried to think of clever titles that reflected my (hopeful) new slim and sophisticated Melbourne persona and also showed that I was on a health and weight-loss journey, but everything I came up with sounded like a novel you'd find in a bargain bin. Maybe my old boss was right – I was fooling myself if I thought I could ever be a writer.

A waiter came over to wipe the table next to me and noticed my empty glass. 'Would you like another one?' he asked.

'Yes, please,' I said, mentally calculating whether I had enough cash on me for a second coffee.

'What were you having? A latte?'

I nodded. 'Skinny latte.'

If I had been in a cartoon, a light bulb would have appeared over my head.

That night I created a blog named 'Skinny Latte: The adventures of a weight watcher'. Like many blogs in 2005, it had a bright colour scheme, photos that weren't sized properly and a badly organised sidebar, but it was my new online home and I was quietly thrilled with it. Being a completely non-technical person, I had no idea what I was doing in the back-end but luckily it was fairly idiot proof. In my first post, I spilled out my story about being overweight at school, the starving and manic exercising to fit into my wedding dress nearly four years earlier, the overeating, the weekends of bingeing and sitting idle. To my great surprise, I didn't feel sad when I recounted those dark days to this unknown internet void. Life would never be like that again, I was certain.

I finally got up the courage to leave a comment on my favourite blogs too – those of M and Mary in Sydney, Emily in New Zealand, and another woman in Queensland. It was slightly awkward at first – after all, I had known these women quite intimately for the last few months, meeting them in the online equivalent of a coffee-house every day, but they had no idea I even existed.

I'm not sure what I was expecting from the blog but I wasn't expecting what actually did happen. The comments I left for other bloggers led them to my site, which in turn prompted them to announce to their readers that there was a new kid in town, which led to more and more traffic and readers as the days and weeks went by. Back in those days, I had no idea about stat counters and visitor tracking; I merely measured everything by the number of comments. I think it's established that comments are no longer the main currency of blogging, as there are far more ways to interact with your readers now, but back then the comments were how we all got to know each other. They were like a trail of point-friendly crumbs to a low-fat gingerbread house. Slowly I followed the trail that led from my blog comments out to others who were in the same boat, · and connections began to be made. With every post, I got more and more comments and 'follows'. For someone who had never been part of a crowd before, and certainly never popular, this was very exciting and, if I'm honest, addictive.

I loved blogging. I wrote the truth as I understood it at the time, with little thought for who might be reading, and while my honesty struck a chord with many, it made me vulnerable in other ways as time went on. However, at the beginning, blogging felt like a secret club, a friendly community of kindred spirits. I felt safe, like I could say whatever was on my mind. I felt supported and understood. It gave me visibility and motivation to keep going, as I was worried that, without a social circle in Melbourne, I might reach for my old friend chocolate cake to keep me company. I needn't have worried – leaving Hobart had not been the soul-shattering and lonely experience I had always feared it would be. I was out of my comfort zone and I missed my family and friends very much but I felt so alive, in a way that I'd never felt before.

I relished the full stretches of day ahead of me when Glenn left for work every morning. I often filled them with trips to the library to collect piles of new books I'd wanted to read for years. We lived in Melbourne's outer north-west and weren't within easy walking distance of public transport so sometimes I joined Glenn on his drive to work, which was closer to the city, and took the tram down into the heart of central Melbourne, spending the day wandering the city, learning it, tracking, negotiating. I wandered through shops full of gorgeous things, none of which I could afford to buy now that I wasn't working. Everyone looked so sophisticated in Melbourne; so many black dresses, well-cut coats and red lipstick. I didn't quite fit that persona yet – I would be lucky if I'd be able to get a haircut every six months. That was something that was bothering me a little: for all my new-found freedom I was now more under the thumb financially than I wanted to be. But how could I be melancholy in this glorious city? I adored Flinders Lane and the City Library, where I usually spent a good part of my days. There were numerous narrow side streets and hidden cobblestoned alleyways in that part of the city and I wandered them all, utterly enchanted. Sometimes I would just hop on trams and see where they took me. I ended up in Brunswick Street one afternoon and browsed through luxurious stationery shops and eclectic fashion boutiques, delighting in the vibrant and funky street art, the smell of coffee and pastries, the budding blossoms on the trees, the trams snaking along the tracks on the road.

I did want to make some new friends, however, and I began to wonder whether there was anyone reading my blog who lived in Melbourne. Ashley's was one of the weight-loss blogs I was now reading daily. She was a few years younger than me, newly married, and studying social work. Her blog entries pulsed with energy; every post was about a gym workout, a new recipe she had cooked, the adventures she and her husband, John, got up to – he was a musician so they seemed to be out doing interesting things all the time. Reading her posts, I was filled with affection for her, and we regularly left comments for each other. One day I read in her latest post that she had shopped for fruit and vegetables at the South

Melbourne Market. My eyes opened wide. She lived in Melbourne! I was so excited. Would I be brave enough to actually suggest meeting someone from the blogs in real life? What if she thought I was a stalker? It was 2005, after all, and the internet was still considered a bit of a dodgy place. So, rather than get too excited at the prospect of a real-life friend I ended up just leaving a comment on that post. Barely a few minutes later, there was a reply from Ashley. *Phil! You've just moved to Melbourne, right? Why don't you come with me to the market next week? I'd love to meet you!* I was ecstatic.

Three days later, I was in South Melbourne, walking up the street to meet Ashley at the market. Glenn had insisted on driving me there, as he was a bit worried about me meeting someone from the internet face to face. He was going to a movie at Crown Casino while Ashley and I wandered around the market. If she turned out to be a psycho, Glenn said, he would have his phone on silent but it would still vibrate. I laughed but it was also nice that he was looking out for me.

I knew it was Ashley the moment I clapped eyes on her. Her hair was auburn, with a few highlights of electric red. She had it swept up on her head in knots. Her nose and cheeks were scattered with freckles and when she saw me approach, a smile lit up her face. I wasn't sure whether a hug would be out of place but Ashley bounded over and gave me a squeeze. 'Hi!' she squealed.

I was instantly at ease. How was it possible that we were only meeting for the first time? We chatted and walked around the snaky aisles of the market, the air rich and pungent with coffee beans, fresh flowers and sandalwood soap. Ashley was steering me towards a particularly bustling part of the market where, the closer we got, I could see a queue of people. The air was fragrant with a tempting, savoury smell.

'If you've never had one, you've got to,' said Ashley as we joined the queue.

'What is it?' I asked, embarrassed by my lack of knowledge.

'Are you kidding?! I've been saving my points all day for this! It's a steamed South Melbourne Market dim sim!'

After watching the stallholders dole out dim sims to the eager market-goers, we finally got ours and found a little table. 'This is heaven in a paper bag,' said Ashley, sitting down. She was right. I savoured the fluffy and perfectly steamed dim sim, dipping it into the puddle of treacly soy sauce in the bag in between bites.

'Oh wow, I could eat a hundred of them!' I laughed as I licked the thick salty sauce off my fingers.

Ashley grinned. 'Three points each!'

We didn't speak much, only emitting an occasional moan of pleasure while we enjoyed every mouthful of our sole indulgence. It was still sinking in for me that I only needed to eat one of something to be satisfied. With half-moons of soy sauce under our fingernails, Ashley and I continued wandering around the market until many of the stalls were starting to close up. I was gazing longingly at the trays of tomatoes they were selling off for two dollars a piece when my mobile beeped with a text message from Glenn.

So, is she a psycho, or are you ok and want to hang out a bit longer?

We ended up going to Richmond, where Ashley's husband was already at a pub. Glenn was persuaded to come along too and although I was initially worried he would just talk cricket or tell terrible jokes, he was in surprisingly good form. I sipped a glass of Western Australian sauvignon blanc, chilled to perfection, and sat in the beer garden with my husband and new friends at my side, an entire world away from what life had been only a year ago. I remember how bright and warm the sunshine was that day, the buzz of the young crowds in the Richmond streets, how much happy energy there was everywhere. It tingled through me like electricity. I'd never thought of joy being something you felt physically in your body, but having started to make friends with this five-foot-ten frame of mine, I was tuning in and realising I was actually *feeling* young, alive and excited by life.

Highs, lows and plateaus

My fat clothes were now laughably big but my thin clothes were not yet a good enough fit for me to feel comfortable wearing them in public. These were jeans, dresses and skirts given to me by my much slimmer younger sister Liz, who, despite having had a baby the year before and now having another on the way, was still smaller than me. I tried them on periodically and each button that did up felt like a victory, even if I'd had to hold my breath while doing so.

The scales hadn't budged for weeks, despite still tracking points religiously and exercising every day without fail. Nearly all the weight-loss bloggers I read were raving about running so, fed up with my third stagnant week in a row, I laced up my sneakers one morning after Glenn had left for work and decided to see if I could just run for five minutes. I hadn't been a bad sprinter as a kid, usually winning ribbons in races at school athletics carnivals. I'd even been picked for the cross-country team in Year 7 but had been quietly relieved when I was diagnosed with mild asthma, which got me out of it. Why had I hated exercise so much? Why had I been so afraid of running? I didn't know where the damage had been done but I wanted to undo it. I enjoyed being active now and had often seen women jogging along the street, or in a park, and they looked so elegant and effortless. How hard could it be?

I power walked to the end of my road to warm up, then broke into a jog once I reached the bushland by the creek that led up towards the main shopping hub of the area we lived in. It felt good at first; my breathing was faster but I felt focused, only looking at the path ahead. Wow, this was easy! But within seconds, my legs started to ache and my breathing intensified. I felt sweat dripping down my face. I was sure I was going to keel over any second. I looked at my watch, convinced I was so exhausted because the five minutes were nearly up, but was gutted to realise it hadn't even been sixty seconds! How unfit was I, if I couldn't even run for a measly five minutes? I honestly didn't think I could go on, but my pride was forcing me to put one foot in front of the other, even though everything ached and I felt like I was going to vomit up a lung. Finally 8.54 a.m. appeared on my watch and I could walk for a while.

Then it started to rain, spilling down in heavy sheets, so in order to get home quickly, I started running again, this time for two minutes, then a break, then another two minutes, then another break. The rain felt incredible on my hot, sweaty face. During my walking breaks, I tried to psych myself up. 'Come on,' I muttered to myself between desperate breaths. 'You're doing this because you need to challenge yourself. The weight will never come off if you don't work hard. Keep going. It will get easier.' I puffed and shuffled along the trail by the creek, blinking furiously to keep the rain and sweat out of my eyes.

I got home from that run feeling absolutely incredible. Like so many things in my life recently, feeling determined and drawing on all these inner resources I didn't know I had was an unfamiliar but wonderful experience. Getting out of my comfort zone was my new addiction. It gave me a high and a rush that food never had. Everything I'd ever wanted to achieve with my life no longer felt impossible. I had proof in front of me that if I tried, I would find out what I was capable of. It was an amazing feeling that I clung to with all my might.

*

The blog continued to be my outlet and my way to meet people in Melbourne. Around this time I made two more wonderful blogging friends. Meredith was about my age, also trying to shift the kilos. As we had been reading each other's blogs for a few months, we knew a lot about each other by the time we met in person. Meredith was a Melbourne girl born and bred, quite shy but very sweet and keen to include me in her life. It was obvious she admired me very much and was in great awe of my weight-loss success so far. She constantly told me how inspiring I was, how seeing me getting closer to my goal was spurring her on too. She had tried and failed to lose weight many times, she said, and thanks to me she thought it was finally going to happen for her. Rather than ringing any alarm bells, this effusiveness just made me feel very special and I was determined to be the best, most inspiring friend possible.

The other friend I made was a woman in her thirties named Gillian, who lived a few hours out of Melbourne. We exchanged emails for a while and then one night, having given her my phone number, she rang me and we talked on the phone for hours, like we were old friends. We talked regularly after that and she even came down to Melbourne one weekend to meet me. She seemed, almost immediately, to fill an older sister role in my life. Like Meredith, Gillian had been trying to lose weight for some time and believed that getting some external accountability was the way forward. She had even auditioned for the next series of *The Biggest Loser*. She was ballsy, bubbly and sophisticated and I loved her company. It was so strange, looking back, how readily I trusted these people and how quickly they became a part of my life. It didn't occur to me for a minute to be cautious.

Glenn and I spent Christmas of 2005 in New Zealand. It was our first overseas trip together and the first time I had ever left Australia, so it felt momentous to say the least. Christmas 2004 had been a bit of a disaster, and we had resolved to make the next one really special. I was now in the habit of sticking to my resolutions, so there we were, spending Christmas in New Zealand and it was the happiest one I'd had for years. We flew into Wellington and hired a car to drive to Auckland, stopping in Taupo and Rotorua on the way. Auckland was a charming city, serene and calm on Christmas Day. In the morning we went to a class at the flagship Les Mills gym, something I would never have done on holiday before, let alone on Christmas Day, and then enjoyed a buffet lunch at the

Sky Tower. We even met up with a few bloggers, which had blown my mind ever so slightly. We met Lee-Anne in Rotorua and Emily and her husband, Jonny, in Auckland; they were all friendly and welcoming and everything I thought they would be. When I thought about how different life had been just one year earlier, I couldn't quite believe it. It was such a happy time. Glenn and I had many wonderful talks on this holiday and spent some real quality time together, exploring the cities, going out for meals, playing cards with a bottle of wine in our hotel room of an evening. I felt so close to him. This was exactly what I wanted my life to be – full of adventure and new experiences, shared with someone I loved.

*

Life took a bit of a strange turn once we came back from New Zealand. The initial excitement of moving to Melbourne began to wear off as talk moved to a subject that had always been tricky in our relationship – money. Glenn said he wanted me to get a job again as he was concerned about our financial situation. He intimated that he was no longer happy about me taking the year off to study, as we'd discussed, because it would mean dipping into our savings. I didn't really understand why he'd had such a change of heart – he knew this was something I wanted to do, that it was a positive step forward for me and for us. More to the point, I had worked to support us in the past and I had thought this was going to be my turn to be supported.

My assertiveness muscles were still very young and they wore out quickly. I lost heart as the conversation continued. Eventually I agreed to defer my university place until the next year and look for a job. But unlike the me of a few years earlier, I was conscious I was sacrificing myself and what I wanted to do. It wasn't sitting well this time because I knew it didn't have to be this way. I now had evidence that if I set goals and went after them, I could achieve them. I could change things in my life I wasn't happy about. So why had I just agreed to do something I didn't want to do – again? The voice that had cried out to me in the shopping centre car park in Hobart had been getting louder and louder. In my journal, I described this time as 'trying to tune in to an out-of-reach radio station. I know it's there and I can hear fleeting sentences, many different voices scattered on the wind blowing through my mind – but I can't get the signal right. I can't tune in.'

I couldn't say for sure this was when my relationship with Glenn changed, but things certainly felt different after that conversation. I wasn't willing to do whatever it took to keep him happy any more. I was tired of our life being structured around only his priorities. It was starting to dawn on me that my happiness wasn't as important to him as his was to me, and perhaps it never really had been. I remembered, leading up to the wedding four years earlier, going alone to the church to meet the minister who was going to marry us. Glenn had refused to miss his cricket club meeting, which was on the same night, and because neither meeting could be moved, he told me I had to go by myself. I wondered whether that was the moment I should have seen into the future I was now living in. A life where I regularly had to accept a lesser version of what I wanted, and where the most important thing in Glenn's life was not, and probably never would be, me.

*

71

After cracking my plateau in November the scales had stalled again. I couldn't believe how close I was to the final hurdle – only 6 kilograms from my goal weight – and yet I was still so far. Glenn, however, was still dropping the kilos and Ashley, also a few kilograms away from goal, was more determined and motivated than ever, which made me a little despondent but also determined to keep up with them and crack the barrier somehow. But after a particularly miserable rainy January afternoon alone in the house, I found myself grabbing the rest of the low-fat ice-cream from the freezer, smashing the rest of my Christmas chocolates into it – Cherry Ripes, Ferrero Rochers, Peppermint Crisps – and eating it on the couch. It sat like a cold stone in me afterwards. I had felt a little better while eating it, but once I had the empty bowl in front of me, I was back to square one. I went to the computer and wrote.

> Why am I doing this to myself? Why am I going back to the old habits when I have healthy new ones that make me feel so much better? I received some beautiful emails over the weekend from some people who have read my blog, and I was so honoured and flattered by their words – and after my ice-cream binge I felt like such a fraud.
>
> The fact that I am having these thoughts after these setbacks shows how far I've come. The old Phil would not have thought twice about an ice-cream binge – it was a regular thing for her. The fact that I am questioning why I did it, and how I can avoid it in future, says a lot about how far I've come. I must seem like

such a hypocrite to you all, after all my hoo-hah about why I'm still doing this and how much I love my life now, how anything is possible. I still believe all those things, but my problem at the moment is that I seem to oscillate between being this superwoman-type woman who says, 'I can do it!' and this sad little thing who wallows in self-pity, who isn't sure who she is, what she wants or where she belongs.

Even with all the self-pity, I know very well there is no way I'm going to go back to where I was a year ago. The reason I have stuck with it, through all the hard times and disappointments, is because I didn't want to be like that any more.

I just have to keep going, no matter how hard it is, no matter how slow the progress. Because I have to. This is how I live life now. There's no going back. If I walk away from it now, if I give up now, then I've learned nothing.

Despite knowing things had shifted a little between us, and being too scared to pull at that thread, Glenn and I were both making more of an effort to do the unexpected and break the routine, to give our relationship the chance to breathe – the way you'd open windows to air out an abandoned house. Our fourth wedding anniversary was the happiest one we'd had. One night a few weeks later, we had finished dinner and Glenn suddenly grabbed the car keys and told me we were going out for dessert. We drove to St Kilda, one of my favourite parts of Melbourne, and we strolled hand in hand along Acland Street, weaving in and out of the Saturday night crowds. In my new (and already loose) size 12 sundress and under Glenn's admiring gaze, I felt beautiful. The night air was warm and I felt deliriously happy. We shared a bowl of ripe, fragrant strawberries with a small scoop of creamy gelato on top and I remember the tender way he looked at me as we ate them. It was like we were in our own private universe. I wanted to bottle the moment. When we arrived home, Glenn whisked me into his arms and carried me inside, something he had only done once before, many years earlier. That night I felt overwhelmed with love for him, confident that whatever feelings of dissatisfaction I may have had about our life, it wasn't our relationship that was the problem. I just needed to get over myself. He was sweet, he was kind; he was worthy of my adoration and trust. All was well.

The next week, I started my new job in the city and, despite everything, was thrilled to be back in the thick of it again. I got home on my first day, tired but exhilarated, to some unexpected news. Glenn was in trouble at his job. He came home that night uncharacteristically quiet. The story he gave me was that a colleague had falsely accused him of misconduct. It didn't even occur to me that if that were true, Glenn would have been livid, unable to be calmed at the injustice of it. Instead, he was silent, brooding and scared. But I accepted his version of events. I had no reason not to believe him.

Around 5 o'clock the next morning, Glenn gently shook me awake and told me he hadn't slept all night. I didn't understand – if he had done nothing wrong, why was he so worried?

'I didn't tell you everything,' he said quietly.

As the sky grew light, he told me what had really happened and it became clear to me this would have serious consequences. Glenn wouldn't get out of this with his job intact. I didn't know what to think, say or do. If my rose-coloured glasses had been slipping off for the past few months, they had now smashed into a thousand pieces.

Glenn, on the other hand, was in pure denial. He seemed to think everything would be okay. He might get let off with a warning. I was starting to realise the warning had come long ago – and we had both ignored it.

To cut a long story short, Glenn was dismissed. It had all happened so quickly, the reality of it was slow to set in. One minute life was heading in a certain direction and the next, everything had been dismantled and we were left with pieces of our old life in our hands, not sure how to put them back together. Everything we had worked for over the past five years was now up in smoke. All I wanted was to get in a time machine and go back just a few days, to the life I knew we had now lost.

The next day, Glenn announced that he wanted to go to Hobart to see his family for a few days, maybe a week. I didn't argue, but having just started a job and with only one income coming in, I couldn't go along. My wonderful parents, their voices full of concern, kindly offered to pay for a flight for me, but I declined. I wanted to be away from Glenn, just for a day, to breathe. To let out all the sadness, anger and frustration that I hadn't dared express to him, to figure out what came next. Right now, in between pretending to be strong, pretending to understand and pretending to be positive, the truth was I was terrified and furious. The future was no longer clear. I had no idea what would happen next, I just knew it wouldn't be good.

After driving Glenn to the airport, I wandered through our empty house, taking in the dusty floors I hadn't had the energy to clean over the past week and the boxes still not unpacked despite moving in nearly six months earlier. I was not moved to open them, unpack them, put any object in a permanent place.

I felt my appetite slowly returning – I'd barely eaten a bowl of soup over the past week – but I ate only what I wanted. Fresh, vibrant salads with peppery rocket from my garden, marinated Persian feta from the Queen Victoria Market and the last ripe tomatoes of summer; pieces of toast carved from a loaf of pecan and fig bread. I opened a bottle of red wine. I wasn't used to all this solitude, but it was incredibly freeing. On my first night alone in the bed, without Glenn, I stretched out like a starfish. I liked the feeling of the empty space that wasn't taken up by someone else.

Apart from my family, I hadn't told anyone what had happened. I wanted to conceal the unhappy truth for as long as possible, which ended up only being until the next morning, when Meredith rang to say hello. I spoke to her briefly, giving a skeletal version of the story. Concerned, she came over the next evening to keep me company, bringing scrapbooks and girly movies, and I made us a low-point laksa for dinner. It was comforting to have her there.

The following morning, Anne's boyfriend, Mike, a good friend who also lived in Melbourne, rang to catch up and I told him what had happened. A few hours later, he showed up on my doorstep. 'Let's go for a drive,' he suggested. I didn't have the energy to ask where; I just got in the car. Before I knew it we were at Tullamarine and Anne, more than 10 kilograms lighter too and looking fabulous, was waiting for us at the arrivals kerb. I was gobsmacked and overjoyed my friend had dropped everything to fly to Melbourne to be with me.

Anne and Mike hung out with me that entire weekend, so my projected period of solitude did not eventuate – which in many ways was a relief. We cooked, watched DVDs, went for power walks around the creek. They didn't bring up the uncertainty of my future, and I didn't volunteer much information. It was enough to sit, take things in and know I was supported, that I had friends who cared. Having them with me that weekend meant a great deal. Life without Glenn was not as empty as I had believed it would be. I savoured the spacious bed, the small exotic meals, the peaceful stretches of time that were mine to fill as I liked. I knew that would all be over once he returned.

Goal

A month had passed and Glenn had barely started looking for another job. Things had become tense and bleak between us. I was deeply worried – it looked like it would be a long time before he had work again. Glenn didn't really talk to me about how he felt, and I was too angry and frightened to probe him too much. I tried to motivate him to apply for jobs, but it was hard when he wasn't even accepting what had happened.

'I guess I just won't mention that I was let go,' he reasoned as we tried to discuss it one night.

'You weren't let go.' I gritted my teeth. 'You were *fired*. There's a big difference. Why can't you admit you were in the wrong?'

Of course, confronting him with reality never went down well but I desperately wanted to pull his head out of the sand. I probably wasn't as kind as I could have been but I couldn't tell him what he wanted to hear. Every night as we sat down to eat dinner together I would ask him which jobs he had applied for that day and he would usually change the subject. Despite being home all day, he never seemed to do a great deal. I left for work early each morning and it was rare for me to be back before six-thirty in the evening, when the dishes from breakfast would usually still be on the table. Glenn rarely cooked or cleaned; some days he didn't even shower. The house lay in a dank mess. I encouraged him to look through my many cookbooks so he could have something in his repertoire to make life a bit easier. He occasionally made an effort but overall it was clear I was still expected to do the bulk of the housework, as I had always done. The minute I walked in the door he would insist on having my full attention as he recounted some small, uninteresting episode in his day in great detail, usually involving the plot of a movie he'd watched. Sometimes I would go to the bathroom with a book for twenty minutes, just to get away from him, to have some peace. If something didn't change soon, I didn't know what I was going to do. This was all too familiar.

Five years earlier, in 2001, I had found it hard to get excited about our upcoming wedding because the whole question of how we were actually going to live kept raising its inconvenient head. Glenn had been unemployed since he graduated the year before. It was a tough time but I felt obliged to sort Glenn's life out for him as he was clearly struggling. I helped him apply for jobs and lent him my car so he could drive to Centrelink to collect his Newstart allowance every fortnight. I found it hard to believe that there were no jobs. I would point out 'help wanted' signs in shops and Glenn would dismiss them. Trying to motivate him only upset him. Every time I broached the topic of his job search it usually ended in angry words and tears, from both sides. Was this really love? I wondered. It felt more like rescuing. For months it went on like this. It put a huge strain on our relationship, and looking back I must have made him feel terribly inadequate. Perhaps I was trying to change Glenn into the man I wanted him to be, rather than accepting him for who he really was.

Mum and Dad occasionally asked whether I was happy but I rarely gave them a straight answer. The only person who talked directly to me about it was Paula, my aunt. Paula had always been a bit of a role model for me – she was a very intelligent, motivated and successful woman, who ran her own consultancy. Paula, her husband, James, and my cousins Natalie and Stuart were like a second family to me and I'd spent many happy hours in their home, especially when my cousins were young, as I was their favourite regular babysitter.

I was over there one day dropping off some books for one of Natalie's school projects and Paula pressed me to stay for a coffee. She asked how Glenn's job hunt was going and, embarrassed, I tried to fluff something about how there wasn't much around.

'Philly,' Paula began, using her childhood nickname for me and putting her coffee cup down. 'Are you really happy with Glenn?'

I didn't know what to say. When I'd first met Glenn, two years earlier, I would have answered 'yes' to that question without hesitation. But lately, with less than a year until the wedding, I hated to admit that I wasn't all that happy but didn't understand why. I was young, with great prospects and engaged to someone who loved me. That meant I had it all ... didn't it?

'It's just that,' Paula was obviously trying to choose her words carefully, 'he doesn't seem to be … you know, on your level.' She drifted off, obviously feeling as awkward as I did. She patted my hand but I still didn't say anything.

'I'm sorry, darling,' Paula said. 'I don't want to upset you. I'm just not sure what kind of life you're going to have with Glenn. He doesn't seem to want to do anything with himself, whereas you … you have so much potential. And you're giving it all up – for what? I really think you can do better.'

I looked into my coffee cup, feeling hurt and confused. 'Can I do better?' I said, my voice dull. 'Really?'

'Of course! I'm sure you could have anyone you wanted,' Paula said gently.

Well, I couldn't see a queue forming. I was too invested in this relationship now to even consider the idea that I deserved more. It hadn't even crossed my mind. I wouldn't acknowledge that I preferred to tolerate the less-than-ideal aspects of life with Glenn and sacrifice myself, my dreams and my potential than risk being alone. The woman I am now shakes her head sadly at this memory. Why was I so convinced, at twenty, this was my one shot at true love?

'What kind of wife am I going to be if I can't support him through a rough patch?' I asked. 'I know he's not the most go-getting guy on the planet, but I'm sure he's trying his best.'

Paula looked like she wished she'd never said anything. 'I'm sure he is, darling,' she sighed. 'I'm not saying he's not a good person. I know you love him, but sometimes love isn't enough. You can't live on love. Do you really want a life where you're constantly nagging him to get a job, where you're always worrying about money and having to go without? You're only twenty years old. Is that what you want for yourself? It's not that I think the man needs to be the provider, far from it. But there needs to be equality. From where I'm standing, the two of you are very unbalanced. It's you who is giving everything. All he does is take.'

I'd love to tell you I listened to her but you know that I didn't. I was in too deep by then. Wanting out felt like both a selfish indulgence and a betrayal. As it did now.

*

In the present, in this very depressing deja vu situation, Glenn's job hunt continued to be fruitless, and with every passing day I felt both my sanity and any respect I still had for my husband slowly fading. One night I'd had enough of coming home to a messy house, enough of him not pulling his weight, and told him so. Glenn stalked off to the study and slammed the door. I went in about five minutes later to find him furiously typing away at the computer.

'I'm writing a cover letter. Are you satisfied?' he spat.

I folded my arms and leaned into the doorframe, looking at unread novels on the bookshelf. I longed for the day when I might be able to finish work and come home to relax, rather than return to a battleground with a sulky child masquerading as a grown man.

'I'm not used to you speaking to me like that,' he muttered.

I fought my natural urge to apologise. 'Well, you need to swallow your pride. You're not going to get a manager's job after what's happened. You just need to get *something*. Stack shelves if you have to; it's better than nothing. It's so much easier to get a job when you already have one,' I said, suddenly aware of how pleading my voice sounded.

'For fuck's sake, do you think I'm stupid?'

I didn't say anything. I was exhausted. *Please Glenn*, I willed him. *Please just get another job so I don't have to face the reality of who you really are and everything can go back to how it was. Please. I'll keep pretending.*

'We should never have moved here. If we'd stayed in Hobart this would never have happened.' Glenn was beginning one of his rants. I knew what was coming next.

'That's rubbish,' I said.

'No, it's not. I was happy there. I didn't want you to leave your job and sell our new house. I just went along with it to make you happy.' I knew he was just saying this to make me feel as guilty and inadequate as he did.

'Stop trying to drag me down with you,' I said angrily. 'You fucked up all on your own; it had nothing to do with me!'

Glenn stood up from the computer. 'That's really low.'

I ended up apologising. Glenn was unbearable as it was, but with him actually angry with me the house would descend into the marital equivalent of a hung parliament. I drew on my teenage acting skills and assumed the character I had always played in the marriage up until now: devoted wife, supportive, unquestioning, trusting. It was getting harder and harder to play.

*

I had a six-week full-time contract with the same company I'd worked for in Hobart, whose Melbourne office was in Flinders Street. It was odd, stepping into the past a little, but I wasn't the girl who kept a month's supply of Kit Kats in her drawer any more, and worked with new people who only knew the slim and confident person who was showing up each day. My workmates all ate things like donuts, hot chips and McDonald's hash browns on a daily basis, which they always offered to share and I always (politely) refused. My supervisor eventually asked, 'Don't you eat junk food? You're always eating healthy stuff.' So I told my colleagues what I'd been doing for the past eleven months. They seemed impressed and asked me how big I used to be. I happened to have my tracker in my bag, so I got it out and turned to the page where I'd stuck some particularly bad 'before' photos. I looked very different now. The constant validation I was getting on my blog made me feel like this was something to be proud of, not hide as a dirty secret. The looks on my colleagues' faces were priceless. 'You don't even look like the same person,' my supervisor said.

'Your workmates don't know you as "Bigger Phil", remember,' Meredith said sagely when I met up with her later. 'So far it's all been about surprising people you know, but people meeting you now will think this is just you.' It was an interesting thought.

I did notice, however, that once I shared my bigger, deep-fried past with them the daily junk-food scoffing eased and they made an effort to be a bit healthier in the office. (Strangely, when I eventually left that job, they bought a giant gooey chocolate mud cake to send me off with.)

I had been offered a permanent part-time job at the University of Melbourne that was far closer to what I wanted to be doing with myself: helping to run a research centre, planning and running events, editing and managing publications. Thus, once my contract ended at the other company, I began working two jobs – splitting my working week between the university and my other workplace, as they had also offered me some temporary part-time work. I was pleased to have a decent income coming in and even more pleased that I was out of the house.

While I was moving forward in leaps and bounds with my career in Melbourne, very little had changed for Glenn on the job front. Letters and emails (that I usually wrote for him) were sent, phone calls were made (or so Glenn said) and weeks dragged on. He got some interviews, but the minute he mentioned the circumstances of leaving his last job, the interview would be over. Glenn eventually went to see an employment consultant, who suggested he not bring it up in interviews unless directly asked. They also said he needed to present himself better and suggested he invest in a new suit, as the only one he had was the one he'd bought for his last round of job interviews five years earlier – and he had lost nearly 30 kilograms since then. We went to Myer that weekend, bought a new suit, and had a coffee afterwards. I watched people walking past us as we sipped our drinks and saw them watching us also. I felt happy for a brief moment, knowing that to the outside world we looked like any other couple out for coffee on a Saturday. No one would ever have guessed the turmoil and the relentless guilt I was living with. The truth was, I was furious at Glenn. I couldn't believe he had done something so stupid and now, because of that, we were in this mess. I wanted him to pick himself up and get the hell back on the straight and narrow because, if he didn't, I wasn't sure how much longer I could go on. But looking back, I can see why he was so resistant. The balance of power had shifted in our marriage and now the only thing he had over me was this. He was used to being in charge, so of course he was going to fight me.

'Did you hear back from the Flight Centre job?' I asked, running my spoon along the inside of my latte glass. This was the first job Glenn had got to the second round of interviews for and it was looking promising.

'Yeah, they called yesterday,' Glenn's voice sounded full of anticipation and my heart leaped, thinking it would be good news at last. 'And I was one of the four —'

My face remembered how to smile. *Oh, please let this be the one, please let this be over,* I thought.

'— who missed out.' Glenn's voice returned to its glum timbre. He'd been trying to be funny, to trick me.

I expelled a breath, trying to stay calm. 'Do you think this is some kind of joke?' I snapped. He sat there, looking so sad. I felt guilty. I was clearly asking too much of him, when life was already so difficult. It was my fault. I had to try harder.

*

The only thing that gave me any pleasure during this time was my smaller, fitter body. As I inched closer to my goal weight, the readership of my blog increased daily, from all over Australia and the world. I even got recognised by readers in Melbourne a couple of times, which gave me a giddy thrill. I wrote upbeat blog entries about my progress with running, as I was now able to run in bursts of ten minutes or more; my latest healthy food discoveries and low-point recipes; and my general delight about life in Melbourne, which despite everything, I still loved and found to be such an exciting vibrant place. It's estimated that blogs and social media only show around 10 per cent of the writer/curator's real life, and this was never more true than with my blog at this time. It's very easy to edit your life down to the shiniest parts, the only parts you're prepared to face and let others see. I don't think my readers were any the wiser about what was really going on. It wasn't that I didn't want to talk about it; every time I logged in, I longed to write about what was happening. The people who read my blog were so supportive and left me such kind, uplifting comments, so I was sure they would comfort me and have good perspectives on the subject. But I knew it was best to keep this out of the spotlight for the time being. I could barely talk about it with people in my real life.

By April, things hadn't improved so I brought up the idea of going to marriage counselling.

'Neither of us is happy, Glenn,' I said as I perched nervously on the edge of the couch. 'You losing your job has really changed things. I think we need to talk about it with someone. We need some help to get through this.'

It had gone beyond the point where I could just have a quiet word to Mum, my sisters or Anne on the phone and blow off a bit of steam about Glenn's sullen and stubborn behaviour, his increasing inability to keep his temper, his general negative outlook and his refusal to take responsibility for his actions. Every day, he acted as though he had chosen to leave his job rather than acknowledging what had actually happened, which made it impossible for us to move forward as a couple.

As I expected, he refused to go to counselling. 'I don't think things are that bad,' he said. 'Nothing's changed.'

For a marriage in trouble to even have a remote chance of being saved, both parties need to want it to work. But at that moment, I was standing alone, not sure what I was even fighting for.

*

Life continued to drag on like this and Glenn remained oblivious to my growing distance from him. If he was worried about our marriage, he hid it well. I tried not to start too many fights and swallowed my frustrations as often as I could. There was no joy or laughter in our home any more. Our life together seemed so empty when I looked around at the world, at my friends' lives, and at my dreams, long faded, of what my life would be like – both as a married woman and as a vibrant person who wasn't yet twenty-five. I had to accept this was a life I had chosen, whether I liked it or not. This realisation made me feel even worse, like I should be trying harder to save this relationship. I was married to the guy; I couldn't just walk out – could I?

One day at my university job, one of the conference managers was putting together a delegate pack for an upcoming event and wanted me to test out some pens.

'You like to write, don't you?' my colleague asked. 'You'll be able to give me a good idea of ink flow and wrist comfort!'

I tested these pens, writing things on sticky notes. At first I just drew my signature, but before I knew it I found myself writing out everything that was in my heart, every scrap of confusion and fear and guilt.

I don't think I love Glenn any more.

He doesn't seem to think anything has changed.

Maybe the novelty is finally wearing off. Maybe we weren't destined to be together.

I miss the old Glenn.

He doesn't understand because, to him, nothing has changed.

I feel so guilty. It's for better or for worse, not for better or until the road gets rocky. But I can't even see the road any more.

Later that afternoon, I made an appointment with a free counselling service at my workplace. Glenn mightn't think we needed help, but I did. I was tired of starting every day with a heavy feeling in my heart, not seeing an end in sight to this drudgery, this guilt, this misery, of having to live with someone you knew you didn't feel the same about any more. It was all such a mess. When I thought about having to explain everything I felt overcome with exhaustion. I just wanted someone to tell me what to do.

The counsellor assigned to me introduced herself as Iris, and I tried to smile as I shook her dry hand, sat down and explained as briefly as I could why I had come there.

Iris pushed her wiry glasses back. 'How do you feel things have changed?'

That was the thing. Glenn was actually right about something: nothing had really changed. It was just that I was finally able to see it for what it was – a life I didn't want to live and a man I didn't want to be tied down to any more. And yet I had wanted both him and this life quite desperately – once. And because of that past self, that crazy, lonely, needy past self, I felt I needed to be there, in that counsellor's office, fighting for my marriage even though my heart was telling me to go.

Iris, to my frustration, did not offer the practical advice I had come for. Instead, she was very interested in something I said, almost as an afterthought – that I had been noticing other men lately, seen them notice me in return, and was curious about what it would be like to be with someone else.

'Well, that's very symbolic of what's lacking in your marriage,' Iris said. 'You know, feeling wanted, feeling excited. It's an opportunity for you to forget about everything that's been getting you down, which is why you're finding it so appealing.'

I didn't understand why she'd latched on to this. It's not like I'd had opportunities to do anything; I'd only made eye contact with other men, not embarked on an affair! But she went on about this for a while and so it wasn't quite the hour of enlightenment I had been hoping for. Iris recommended Glenn and I seek relationship counselling and I explained he had already dismissed the idea. I had actually brought it up again the other day, I told her, but when Glenn realised that the local branch of Relationships Australia charged seventy dollars a session, he wasn't so keen on the idea. Glenn wasn't a man who put his hand in his pockets very often, not even to save his marriage. In fairness to him, I too was starting to think no amount of money would fix us.

Iris said if that was the case, all I could do was a stocktake of my life, as painful as it might be, and decide what sort of future I wanted, and then how my relationship with Glenn would fit in with that, rather than the other way around, as I had been doing for the past seven years.

'I can help you draw things out and make sense of how you're feeling,' Iris said plainly, 'but it's up to you to come to your own conclusions.'

Afterwards I walked back to my office, tightening my too-big jacket around me against the icy late-autumn breeze, feeling more lost than ever.

*

A few nights later, I needed to work late so I called Glenn at four to tell him that I would have to stay until about seven, therefore probably not getting back to the train station until after eight. Could he please cook dinner and have it ready for when I got home?

Silence. 'What am I going to make?' he asked sulkily.

'I don't know. I don't remember what we've got in,' I replied, annoyed that he needed me to walk him through such a simple request. 'I don't mind, really, just make something with whatever's in the cupboard; that'll be fine.' I rang off and went back to my work.

I got back to the train station just after eight as anticipated and was met with a loaded silence in the car, a furious Glenn at the wheel.

'What's wrong?' I asked with caution.

'You asking me to cook dinner, that's what,' Glenn snapped, his jaw locked in anger as he turned out of the station parking lot.

I felt tense with irritation. 'Why? I've been working late. You've been at home all day.'

'Well, we haven't been grocery shopping this week, so there was hardly anything left. Everything I know how to cook we didn't have the ingredients for.'

'We live a five-minute walk from a supermarket.' I was trying to stay calm. 'You could have gone and got whatever you needed.'

It didn't matter what I said; Glenn believed my asking him to cook dinner for us that evening was completely unreasonable. To add fuel to the fire, when Glenn had finally started to cobble something together he had burned his finger, which was now causing him considerable pain and distress.

'From now on, if I have to cook dinner, I want at least twenty-four hours' notice,' he said.

Poor Glenn. How could I have expected a man who had been unemployed for nearly three months, who sat at home and did very little with his day, apart from watching the midday movie, to cook the evening meal? The injustice of it! It was so ridiculous I started laughing.

'You want twenty-four hours' notice to cook dinner?' I repeated incredulously. 'Are you serious?!'

Glenn went on a rampage. It was all my fault – I worked late too much; I was working two jobs and was never home any more; I hadn't given him enough notice; I had monopolised the kitchen and the cooking for our whole marriage and had never given him a chance to shine.

'How dare you be so disrespectful!' he stormed. 'Do you have any idea how hard the last few months have been for me?'

I had no fight left. I sat silently as we got closer to the house. I knew he was waiting for an apology. In the past, in situations like this (and there had been many of them, mostly over card games) I would usually back down and tell myself, 'Just be the bigger person and apologise, and then you can forget about it.' I didn't want to do that any more. I was tired of always having to give in. It was about time Glenn knew I was a woman to be reckoned with. I wanted some respect. I also wanted to be married to a man who didn't behave like a three-year-old. If I wanted to be married at all.

We finally got home. I managed to salvage the dinner, gave Glenn an icepack for his finger, and we sat down to eat the soup, which tasted burned.

'Is it good? Do you like it? Didn't I do a great job?' Glenn asked every three minutes, desperately wanting praise.

I could barely swallow it.

*

That night propelled us into a space where we had no choice but to talk about the battleground our marriage had become. In the days that followed we had some fairly frank talks about the state of our relationship, initiated by me, and Glenn finally admitted that he wasn't all that happy either. We discussed the possibility that giving each other space to reclaim our own identities, rather than being in each other's pockets as we had been for almost seven years, might ease things. Perhaps we needed some time apart?

We didn't agree on anything; these scary concepts were just floated and left hanging as the conversation wound down and we both tried to press on. As his job search continued to be fruitless, Glenn told me he was considering joining the armed forces, which would likely mean leaving Melbourne if he was accepted. That was the last thing I wanted to do, but he told me he wouldn't expect me to come with him. What did that mean then? I wondered. Every day it seemed there was another curveball thrown into this already crowded tennis court. I was whacking them away as fast I could but I was slowly wearing down. It wasn't love that was keeping me there, with him, in that house. It was guilt.

Redemption was occasionally offered as the nights grew darker and we marched towards winter. Sometimes Glenn would pick me up late from the train station, and the car would be filled with the delicious smells of garlic naan and lamb pasanda, which he had ordered and picked up so I wouldn't have to cook. One day I came home and found a small bottle of my favourite perfume on my side of the bed. On a Sunday stroll around Highpoint shopping centre I expressed admiration for an expensive winter coat, and Glenn took it up to the counter and paid for it without a word, telling me it could be my birthday present.

I couldn't deny I liked this side of him but I suspected that his generosity had fear at its core. By showering me with gifts and giving me the thoughtful attention I'd always craved, he was effectively bargaining with me not to leave.

Glenn was also still managing the household finances and I was starting to resent this, given that I was the only one bringing in any income. I wanted more input and he took this very badly. He came from a very traditional family and having a woman as the sole provider was probably something he couldn't get his head around, which would explain his aggression and constant disparagement of my achievements. In Hobart I had only been interested in him and meeting his needs. I was blossoming in Melbourne and Glenn didn't seem happy about it. I can understand that – just as the sweet guy I'd married had disappeared, the endlessly patient, placating and eager-to-please girl he'd married no longer existed either. Perhaps he was just as heartbroken as I was.

'Maybe we need to start having separate finances,' Glenn finally said, looking at his shoes.

'Yes, maybe we do,' I admitted. 'I'm tired of working this hard and not even being able to get a haircut. I've worked so hard to lose all this weight too and yet I'm still wearing size 16 clothes that are too big for me. It sucks.'

My words were only met with silence. 'What did you apply for today? Anything?' I asked him.

'No. There wasn't anything good.'

I sighed and Glenn just glared at me. 'Something will come along. I'll get a job,' he snapped. He paused, and then added, '*You* managed it; it can't be that hard.'

I stood up. 'Separate finances it is.'

*

It was nearing the end of April and was coming up to a year since I had stepped on the scales and seen 103.5 kilograms staring back at me. Every week I was diligently weighing in and reporting the results on my blog, but I had hit another plateau. It was the last kilogram that was proving the hardest to lose, weirdly enough, but I had grown bored of pressuring myself. Progress had been made, I knew that, and the scales would catch up eventually. I was well and truly committed to being healthy and fit. The rewards were far greater than anything I had given up in the process. Reaching that magic number on the scales wasn't going to spell the end of this journey for me.

I was proud that I hadn't turned to food to keep the sadness, frustration and guilt about what was happening in my marriage at bay. I felt grateful for the support and accountability of the blogging community, and the wonderful friends I had made from it. I felt so motivated by seeing others succeed and reach their goals, and I was thrilled that I was being held up as a success story too. For the first time in my life I did feel like a success. I had set a goal and I was so close to achieving it. I hadn't given up on the hard days when I'd lost my grip a little; I was learning to keep my all-or-nothing thinking in check. But most of all, what my nearly 30 kilogram weight-loss was proving to me was that if there was something in my life I wasn't happy with, I had the strength and the power to change it.

When Anzac Day dawned, exactly one year since stepping on the scales in my carpeted bathroom in Hobart, I decided to step on them again. Just to compare, one year on.

The dial went straight to 76 kilograms. Bang on. That last pesky kilogram was gone and the scales were proudly declaring I had reached the goal I had set out to achieve. The number that had felt so impossible a year ago. I had stuck to the plan. I hadn't given up. I called Glenn in to check, just in case I was seeing things, but he confirmed it. Goal.

Wow, I did it, I thought.

And if I can do this, maybe I can do anything.

Be careful what you wish for

A few days after I reached goal and after the virtual party that had been held online when I announced my triumphant news on my blog, Glenn and I went down to Hobart to meet our new baby nephew and catch up with my family, who I hadn't seen nearly all year. I was wearing a belt to keep my size 12 jeans up, which was a first.

Despite my putting on a brave face, my mother sensed all was not well.

'Are things okay with you and Glenn, love?' she asked gently when we were finally alone. She had picked me up from coffee with a friend and we were driving home.

I opened my mouth to answer but found I couldn't speak, my voice silenced with tears. I could only shake my head.

Mum looked at me sadly. 'I hope I'm not speaking out of turn, but I get the feeling you're not in love with him any more. Are you?'

'I don't know,' I choked out, the tears now streaming down my face. 'I don't know any more. I'm so confused. I feel so guilty.' Even though I knew I didn't feel the same way about Glenn as I used to, I also felt miserable at the thought of being without him. He was all I'd ever known. I hated the thought of someone else having to learn everything that Glenn already knew, even though how much he really knew about me was questionable.

Mum listened as we headed back to the house, not forcing her opinions on me or telling me what I should do, just letting me talk and sob in the warm comfort of the car, and once the car was parked she held me.

'I only want you to be happy,' Mum said. 'That's all your father and I have ever wanted for you. We thought you married Glenn very young, but I knew you would do it anyway, regardless of what we had to say, and I wanted you to be married with our blessing rather than without it.'

As she spoke, I realised what a noble act of restraint my parents had performed for me. Five years ago they had seen me at the doorstep of an enormous mistake and instead of talking me out of it, they had let me go. Just as when I was learning to walk, they had let me fall. It was the only way I would learn.

Ever since that horrible day in the car park the year before, I had tried to take back control of my life, to eliminate the things that were making me unhappy. On the surface the answers had been easy. Lose weight. Get fit. Move interstate. Spread my wings. Start writing again. Make new friends. As I'd unpicked the stitches of that old life, I couldn't shift the sad, guilty knowledge that there was still one thing weighing me down.

*

The weekend after we got back home, Meredith had a birthday dinner down at the Docklands. We had some drinks while getting ready at the flat she shared with her boyfriend, Justin, and then the three of us caught a cab to the restaurant. Glenn was going to join the party later. I felt resplendent and glowing in my new chocolate-brown silk dress, enjoying the fact it showed off my collarbones, toned arms and tiny waist. It was only my heart that was still heavy.

Meredith's party proved to be great fun. I had always yearned for this kind of life – to be out on a Saturday night with friends instead of on the couch, my mouth furry with sugar, watching the football or some gormless film. A few of Meredith's workmates were there and I enjoyed chatting to them. Most of them were men and I noticed the approving looks they gave me with a lot of pleasure. Glenn barely complimented me any more. In fact, he had never seemed particularly proud to be with me. He once told me, when we'd met all those years ago at ballroom dancing classes, that the general consensus among the young males who went along was that my sister was the more attractive of the two of us, by far, and their nickname for me was 'Claire's ugly sister'. Remembering the dead thud in my chest when he told me that, I felt sorry for that poor girl, who knew very well she wasn't much in the looks department compared with her three athletic, raven-haired sisters, and who just accepted Glenn's tactlessness like she would needles at an acupuncturist. But I certainly didn't feel like the ugly sister these days.

Glenn finally arrived at the restaurant, nodded without inter-est when I told him I'd ordered him a Thai beef salad for dinner (same as me) and ordered a Jack Daniels and Diet Coke. I smiled at him, searching his face for some tenderness that might still be there. He was frowning in the other direction.

'That bloke over there keeps staring at you.' He put an arm around me possessively. 'What's his problem?'

I laughed, trying to keep things light. 'Maybe he thinks your wife is hot,' I said coquettishly.

Glenn *hmphed* into his drink. I took another gulp of my cock-tail. 'I've been getting lots of looks lately, you know. You might have to start working a bit harder,' I teased, giggling.

Glenn simply held up his left hand, where his wedding ring glinted dully in the dim light, thrust it forcefully towards my face, and threw me a look that said, 'I don't think so.'

Another dead thud in my chest. My attempt at humour had clearly hit too close to home, or maybe he just didn't care any more. He had certainly stopped trying. Thankfully our meals arrived and I poked as much chilli-and-lime-soaked beef and salad into my mouth as my churning stomach would allow, cosied up to Meredith and talked to her about more pleasant things, trying to ignore the familiar guilty feeling gnawing away at me. If I couldn't have what I wanted, I would just have to try harder to want what I had.

*

A few weeks later, Glenn had an interview, the first one in a month. I finished work a few hours early and met him afterwards. It had gone well and Glenn looked happier and more relaxed than he had in some time. We caught the train home together and I listened to Glenn talk about the interview and the jokes he had cracked that the interviewers had laughed at. I leaned back in my seat and thought, *Everything will be all right.* We did the grocery shopping on the drive home and we were unpacking them in the kitchen when the phone rang. Glenn raced to answer it and I felt my body ripple with nausea. I hoped this would be the call that would turn everything around.

Glenn came back into the kitchen and his face was a picture of happiness. 'I got the job!' His voice broke on the last word. I threw myself into his arms and felt him lift me off the ground. I buried my face into his neck, breathing the old him back, the old life, the old love. I felt tears sting my eyes and tense breaths fall out of my body.

'That's such wonderful news! Let's go out and celebrate?'

Glenn looked at me. 'No, we just spent a hundred bucks on groceries. We should just eat here.'

And there he was, the old Glenn. I thought the hardship of the last few months might have instilled some humility in him. My heart sank as I realised he hadn't changed at all.

We rang our families with the news and then I made pita-bread pizzas for dinner. *Well, this is what you wanted,* said the voice inside my head as we sat together on the couch later, watching TV. *He's got a job. It's all back to normal now.*

*

My twenty-fifth birthday was a few days later, at the end of May, and despite the state of my marriage, it was one of the happiest birthdays I'd ever had, full of dumplings, cocktails, cake, gelato and good friends. It was the first birthday in my twenties I hadn't marked with a Woolworths chocolate mud cake – to myself. Instead, I wore my size 12 jeans with a belt and felt like Superwoman. The year before I had been heavy and heartbroken, red-faced and double-chinned in every photo; but now I was slender and slim-hipped. I was still heartbroken, but not in the same way. I still somehow believed everything was going to be all right. Glenn and I had even booked another trip to New Zealand together for October. But life yet again whacked me around the face and showed me how, in one fragile second, everything can change.

It was the day after my birthday. Anne was in Melbourne that weekend, and she and Mike came around for dinner and general merriment. We enjoyed a bottle of wine. Mike had brought a Play-Station game with him, which captured Glenn's interest immediately. Always eager for any chance to shine, he loved thrashing people at games and boasting about it afterwards, which tended to take all the fun out of it for everyone else. It was an irritating trait of his I had always tolerated and excused but in actual fact, like nearly every-thing else about him lately, I found it deeply embarrassing.

Glenn lost the game, threw the console down and stormed out in a huff. The three of us laughed, because here was a grown man exercising less self-control than your average two-year-old. I called out, 'It's only a game! Don't be so immature!' and continued laugh-ing from my cross-legged position on the floor. Glenn then came back into the room, glaring at me. This is what struck me – there was time for him to think before he did what he was about to do.

There was no love in his eyes any more. Before I knew what was happening, he had swung his foot back and kicked me.

Time suddenly stood still, like it does in dreams. I remember Anne raising her voice. I didn't say a word; I was simply frozen to the spot. I thought any minute now I would wake up and life would resume as it had been only seconds earlier. But it didn't. Nothing could rewind that moment. Nothing could take it back.

He left the room and I heard the bedroom door slam. Anne and Mike gazed at each other and then at me, full of concern, but none of us spoke until I finally broke the silence.

'I'm so sorry.' Even my voice didn't sound the same.

'What are you apologising for, honey?' asked Anne. I think she was crying. 'You have nothing to be sorry for!'

I now understood the feeling of wanting the earth to open up and swallow you. I was beyond mortified. The awful knowledge that I was married to someone like that, who would lash out at me in front of our friends, filled my heart with shame. Up until that point I had convinced myself our marriage could be saved, that we could get past this. But now, I knew it was over.

Sadly, it was the wake-up call I needed. Despite everything, I had still been putting Glenn first. I had been less patient than he was accustomed to but I had still tolerated his bad behaviour, his temper, his constant disparagement of me and my achievements. I knew things were disintegrating between us, but out of pride, fear of judgement or a sense of loyalty I kept giving him another chance. Despite reaching my goal weight and projecting an aura of confidence out into the world, I still didn't believe I deserved more than what Glenn could offer. I had to wait for something like this to happen before I would give myself permission to go.

Even now, ten years later, I feel ashamed when I remember and talk about that night. There is still a part of me that feels I over-reacted and made a fuss about nothing. But then I remember the shock on my friends' faces and the crying in the bathroom after-wards with the taps turned on so he wouldn't hear me, and I know – whatever it was, it wasn't nothing.

Eventually I went into the bedroom to try to talk to him. Hav-ing had nearly an hour to think about what happened, I thought Glenn would be inconsolable, begging for forgiveness. He wasn't.

'I'm sorry other people saw it,' Glenn said, 'but I'm not sorry I did it. You brought it on yourself. You deserved it. You were so rude and disrespectful to me. I was so embarrassed.'

I finally found my voice. '*You* were so embarrassed?' I exclaimed. 'Am I actually hearing you right? You think what you did was okay?'

'Why did you make me do that to you, Phil? After everything I've done for you for your birthday.' Glenn looked at me mournfully. 'I bought you that dress, that coat, the perfume —'

'Oh, and that gives you the right to kick me, does it?'

'You aren't even taking on board what I'm saying. I can't believe that you won't even try to see this from my point of view. You're always picking on me these days. If you hadn't made me so angry, I wouldn't have done it.'

I took a deep breath. 'Look, I know the last few months have been difficult. I'm sorry that I've lost patience with you and haven't been hiding it, like I usually would. But if you think,' I said slowly, 'in any way, that what you just did to me was okay, then we have a very big problem.'

Actually, we'd had a big problem for a long time. I looked into his face and realised that the only thing I felt was a desire to get as far away from him as I possibly could. But I only went as far as the living room, where Anne and Mike had opened another bottle of wine – it seemed the only thing that would calm all our nerves – and cried, with each of them taking a turn to comfort me. It was a long, awful night.

When I went back into the bedroom a few hours later, the lights were out and Glenn was in the bed, curled up, pretending to be asleep. There was a note on my side of the bed. I took it into the bathroom to read. The note was apologetic but only to a point. Glenn wrote that he felt I had not been as supportive as I could have been over the past few months and that was why he had snapped. But he loved me and wanted to be with me. He reminded me of our recent conversations about separating but said that wasn't what he wanted at all. *I don't want to lose you*, were his last desperate words. I turned on the taps so the noise of running water would drown out my sobs as I sat on the bathroom floor and tore the letter up.

It felt like hours I was in that tiny ensuite bathroom, crying, replaying the horrible scene in my head. Glenn had clearly learned nothing. His complete inability to think before he acted had once again dismantled everything in his life in seconds. And, like his job situation, he was refusing to take responsibility for what he'd done. I think back now and wonder whether it was something else. Perhaps he was actually as unhappy and dissatisfied with our life together as I was, which made him sabotage whatever was still holding us together. Perhaps, in his own way, he too was trying to break free.

I don't remember how or if I slept that night. The next morning things were strained and tense. Anne and Mike had stayed the night in our spare room but we weren't having the fun pancake brunch I had originally planned. Glenn remained quiet but was otherwise carrying on as though nothing had happened. When we all went to the DFO in Essendon later, he held my hand as we wandered around and I didn't pull it out of his reach. Anne remembers things about this that I don't. 'It was as if you'd hit the pause button,' she recalls now. 'You were so embarrassed by what he'd done, but because we were there, you just had to put on a brave face and carry on as normal.' The woman I am now would have exploded at him, or kicked him out of the house. The only explanation I can offer is that, ironically, I didn't want to make a scene.

Later that afternoon, when we were finally alone in the house, it was inevitable we would have to discuss what had happened. By now Glenn had realised I wasn't going to brush this under the carpet, as I had when he'd behaved badly in the past, so while he seemed remorseful on some level, he employed his usual tactic for when he knew he was in the wrong – he denied everything.

'I'd had too much to drink,' he insisted. 'I don't even remember doing it.'

I didn't buy it. I was sure the scene had been replayed in his head as much as it had in mine. As for 'too much to drink', he'd had one glass of wine and two Jack Daniels with Diet Coke (which were more Diet Coke than anything). It was excuse after excuse, and as the conversation went round in circles, he insinuated that I had no right to be angry because he didn't remember what he'd done, that he therefore didn't have to make amends and we should just forget about it.

One voice in my head said, 'Come on, be a big girl, just let it go and move on. I'm sure he didn't mean it,' as it had many times over the years. But another voice, stronger and louder, was saying, 'Go. For God's sake, go. You deserve so much better than this. Run as fast as you can and don't stop running. Your real life is waiting for you. This is not where you stay.'

They were awful, those first few days afterwards. The pain, humiliation and anger at what had happened was so fresh. I barely spoke to him. Desperately missing my family, I booked a flight to Hobart for the weekend. The night before I left, Glenn had the nerve to ask me not to tell my family what he'd done, which suggested he knew he had done something terrible. But the responsibility of sorting out this mess had been placed squarely on my shoulders. Glenn was now apathetic about the whole thing and wanted me to decide what happened next. As far as he was concerned, Saturday night had merely been a big misunderstanding. If I was going to take this as a sign that our marriage was deeply in trouble – even over – then fine. He wasn't fighting for us.

I was met at Hobart Airport first thing on Friday morning by Mum, who sensed immediately that something was wrong. Eventually I told her, Dad and my sisters what had happened and to say they were shocked and appalled is an understatement. We all cried together. The days I spent there were full of comfort and support as I tried to make sense of everything and work out what I should do once I returned to Melbourne. Everyone resisted giving me advice other than that I had to start putting myself first. I couldn't worry about Glenn any more. I only communicated with him via text messages while I was gone. I didn't ask how his first day at his new job had been, and he didn't tell me much, apart from boasting that another woman had checked him out on the tram on his way home.

On my last day in Hobart I caught up with my friend Kristy for coffee and then drove around in the rain for a while, feeling sad every time I saw somewhere that reminded me of Glenn, of a time when we had supposedly been happy. I found myself driving near where my aunt Paula lived and decided to see if she was home. She was.

We sat at her table with mugs of peppermint tea, and I told her what had happened. Her eyes filled with tears. 'He might as well have hit you,' Paula said softly, her voice breaking.

This was something that had been bothering me. He hadn't hit me. Was I just overreacting, using it as a convenient excuse to cut him loose and leave? Or was I stupid if I stayed and tried to work things out? Would he do it again? Deep down I knew the answers to these questions. Glenn had always had a temper and over the years he had occasionally pushed me out of the way when I had annoyed him or screamed at me when he lost a card game – recently, he had even smacked me hard on the bottom as if I were a child when I told him he was irritating me while I was cooking. The events of Saturday night didn't fit into any neat categories of domestic violence but I knew it was the final manifestation of a nasty temper I had tolerated for a long time.

As I sat there, sipping my tea and talking to Paula, Glenn's cold words kept echoing in my mind. You deserved it, it was your fault, you deserved it. Maybe he was right. He hadn't meant to hurt me; I had brought it on myself. Maybe I was just a horrible person who didn't deserve anything better. I was so angry with Glenn but at the same time I was overwhelmed with sadness and felt a strange need to dismiss what he had done, even defend him. He was still, for better or for worse, my husband.

'I know I hurt you that day, when I told you what I thought of him,' Paula said, referring to our conversation of five years earlier. 'I really hoped I was wrong.'

'I wish I'd listened to you,' I said simply.

This time I was well and truly ready for anything Paula had to say but, like everyone else, she was quite reserved with her opinions and said I had to make up my own mind about what happened from here.

'What I will say though, Philly, is the quickest cut is the kindest.' Paula looked at me knowingly. 'Don't drag it out. If you're going to go, then just go.'

*

I arrived at Hobart Airport that chilly Monday night to fly home, sent off with tearful hugs from my worried parents and sisters. Dad had even offered to fly back with me but I knew I needed to face Glenn alone. I walked into the airport lounge only to discover my flight was delayed by four hours. My family had already left after dropping me off, so I was on my own. I sent Glenn a text to tell him about the delay, and bought myself a glass of wine, then a skinny latte (of course), then another glass of wine. I watched couples farewell or greet each other with passion and my heart ached. It actually physically hurt to realise I no longer had that, and that things would never be like that between Glenn and me again.

If I had been confused before flying down, my mind was well and truly in a state of chaos now. Unable to think about anything else, I got out my journal and a pen and decided to do an old-fashioned pros and cons list. On a blank page I wrote, 'Reasons to stay,' and underlined it. I felt I owed Glenn that much: to begin there.

The reasons to stay filled perhaps half a page. They were mostly perfunctory statements like, 'Glenn is very generous, when he wants to be,' 'Glenn is very loving, when he wants to be.' Those five words qualifying characteristics I now felt I deserved to be permanent fixtures in the man I was spending my life with were, despite the wine I had drunk, sobering. Unable to think of anything else, I abandoned the list of reasons to stay. Reasons to go were next. By the time the boarding announcement for my delayed flight came on, I had filled five pages. It was there in front of me, in black and white, that staying was not an option. I had finally admitted to myself that I wanted and deserved far more than Glenn was prepared to offer. Everything in our life together had always been on his terms, when he felt like it. I had always gone along with it because I loved him and wanted him to be happy. Now, *I* wanted to be happy.

The flight touched down in Melbourne just before midnight. Glenn was waiting for me, surprisingly not angry at the delay. We went home and finally talked honestly about what we were going to do. We both wanted out, as it happened. He did most of the talking, very calm and emotionless. As he spoke, I looked over at him, the man who had been the centre of my life for nearly seven years and, just for a split second, the thought of living without him was unbearable. I felt overwhelmed with sorrow, but what I mostly felt was relief.

*

My new life couldn't start straight away. We still had to live together until our rented house, still under a water-tight lease, was re-let. It was hard spending all day dreaming of the exciting things I was at last going to have the freedom to do, and then having to go home to Glenn every evening. He may have been the picture of calm the night I came back from Hobart but over the days and weeks that followed, his facade started fracturing. I stayed out as often as possible. Most nights I deliberately worked until well after seven, and then ate dinner somewhere in the city, wonderful little ethnic cafes where I could get a meal for around five dollars. Occasionally Meredith or Ashley would join me. Otherwise, I would eat and then wander around the City Library or the bookstores in Melbourne Central until they closed. I collected flyers for yoga courses, acting classes, creative writing – anything that might enable me to stay out longer, so I could go another day without dealing with Glenn and the resentment he was directing towards me now the enormity of what lay ahead had hit him.

On a night I was actually home, Glenn called his parents to tell them we were separating. Thanks to the paper-thin walls of that house, I heard the entire conversation. In true Glenn fashion, he did not mention the kicking incident, or his refusal to go to marriage counselling, both now (I had put it to him one last time, for closure if nothing else) and months earlier. He told them the move to Melbourne had really changed me, that I had decided I wanted to focus on my career and that he wasn't good enough for me any more. He made out that I was basically leaving him to fend for himself, interstate, with no friends or support network.

While I was furious listening to this, I wasn't surprised. Glenn had always been economical with the truth, especially when it came to his own shortcomings and, apart from his sister, his family had never particularly warmed to me, so I knew he would work that to his advantage.

It was horrible still living in that house, where everywhere I looked there was rubble of the old life. I had taken down our wedding pictures – in fact, any picture of us together looking happy. I was desperate for another tenant to be found so we could move out and get on with our separate lives. I emailed the landlord every few days to see how things were going and while the replies were always pleasant and hopeful, with every day that passed with no resolution, the tension mounted.

Another evening, I came home from work and went to the computer with the intention of writing my first blog post in weeks. Glenn had been using it, so it was still switched on. I shook the mouse to relieve the screensaver and sat down. I didn't think it was appropriate to share on my blog what had happened but I wasn't sure what else I had to say – the logistics of the separation were all I could think about. I hadn't been watching what I ate, nor had I been running for weeks, and yet even a belt didn't hold my size 12 jeans up any more. I wasn't sure how I was ever going to put this mess into words. Not only was I deeply ashamed my young marriage was over, I was terrified of being judged. I had painted a rosy picture of our marriage on my blog and I knew, without all the private details of what had actually gone on, it would look just like the story Glenn was perpetuating: I had just woken up one day, realised I wasn't fat any more and thought I'd ditch him for something better and more exciting – which was so far from the truth it wasn't funny. But telling the truth right then, in that moment, wasn't an option. I was still processing it.

I looked at the computer screen. A folder was open containing photos of Glenn, topless. In the photos, he was holding an A4 piece of paper with a strange verification code written on it.

'What the fuck?' I said aloud, staring at the screen. Glenn came into the room shortly afterwards, and even though I didn't want to ask about the photos, because I knew he wanted me to, curiosity got the better of me. It turned out they were identity verification photos for a 'website I've registered with'. In other words, chat rooms and internet dating. I was disgusted.

'You could have at least waited until I moved out,' I snapped.

Glenn mumbled something in reply but I was too furious to listen. Why had I ever been worried about being alone? Right then I could think of nothing I wanted more.

There was no point worrying about the future; it was just a matter of getting through one day at a time. Somehow, as the corpse of that marriage was nailed into its coffin, I got through. For the past few months, it had felt like I was drowning. Glenn had been in the deep with me, clinging on to me, both of us sinking. He hadn't been willing or able to save himself. I could have saved him, but in doing so I would have sacrificed myself. I could only save one of us.

I chose me.

PART TWO

Skinny Latte

*'There are only two mistakes one
can make along the road to truth;
not going all the way, and not starting.'*

BUDDHA

The naked Ironman

The last thing I expected to see on my first night in my new home was one of my housemates completely naked. One minute I was lugging a heavy box up the stairs, the next I was staring, speechless, through the open doorway of the bedroom to my right. There was Ironman: tanned, waxed and competition-ready, damp from the shower, applying moisturiser to his firm naked body.

My sharp intake of breath suddenly made Ironman glance away from the mirror and straight at my stunned-mullet expression.

'Shit!' he exclaimed, reaching frantically for his towel.

I quickly turned away and walked round the corner, only to knock myself and the box into the nearby wall.

'Sorry!' I called out, scrambling to get my balance back. 'I'm so sorry!'

I bolted into my new room, closed the door and threw the damn box on the floor, next to the pile of everything else I'd shifted that day. I leaned against the back of the door and found myself laughing. Single life was off to an interesting start.

*

I was now living in Fairfield, a suburb in eastern Melbourne, in a house with two gorgeous men, Ironman and Bomber, both of whom were, as their aliases suggest, incredibly fit athletes. It had taken a while to find them.

When continuing to live with Glenn had finally become more than I could bear, a kind colleague at the university had told me I could stay at her place. She was going to Europe for a month and her house in Greensborough was going to be empty. All that she required was that I water the plants and feed the cats. I had fallen on the vacant house gladly, happy for solitude and silence.

Within a few days of arriving there I caught a terrible flu – Melbourne's winter was frosty and dark, and the cold had seeped into my bones. I crawled into bed at 6.30 every night and slept the sleep of the weary. It had been a very tough couple of weeks. I had been deeply relieved to get away from Glenn but the logistics of it all had been very messy indeed. Half my stuff was still in the old house and I still had to see him and speak to him regularly while the final details of our separate moves were organised. It was strange to be missing him so much and yet every time I saw or spoke to him feel repulsed. I couldn't believe I had ever been in love with him, when he was so rude to me all the time, and so wrapped up in himself. I began to realise he had in fact always been like this but I had been blind to it. And as for missing him, it was the old him I was missing – or maybe it was the old me. It was all very confusing. No wonder I was going to bed so early every night; it was easier to be unconscious.

I finally revealed the news of the separation on the blog at the end of June, once I'd moved out, after encouragement from Meredith, Ashley and a few other blogging friends who were aware of what had happened. I had been so worried about being judged but the comments I got on that post – my longest to date – were nothing but kind and supportive. In fact, many readers came out of the woodwork to comment for the first time and shared their own stories of separation and heartbreak with me. 'I had three kids and was thirty-six before I left,' one told me. 'Stay positive, it gets better.' Well, I was certainly trying to believe that. Some days it was an achievement just to get out of bed. But every day, one foot had to be put in front of the other, and I still needed to find a permanent place to live.

With the help of Hannah, a workmate, I had started scouring Melbourne for an affordable living situation. One of the executive assistants who had been a friendly face at work from day one, Hannah was very well connected when it came to message boards, forums and clubs. She was the sort of person who knew people, who knew someone else, who knew Ironman and Bomber.

I'd looked at rooms in South Yarra, Collingwood, North Fitzroy, Clifton Hill and Brunswick, but every place I could afford either came with questionable stains on the ceiling or carpet, or a strange middle-aged single housemate – perhaps a glimpse into what the future held for me if I didn't get a grip. Finally Hannah came to the rescue with news of a spacious room in a house in Fairfield. Not holding out much hope, I was pleasantly surprised by how friendly Ironman and Bomber were as they showed me around the house. While they pointed out the clean but personality-free kitchen and bathrooms, the deck, backyard and laundry room, I kept thinking, *Two men! Two* hot *men! How is this possible?* It was as if I was nineteen again, or rather, the nineteen-year-old I should have been. My imagination was certainly making up for lost time.

I liked the bedroom – it had built-in wardrobes, a clean ceiling and carpets, and was big enough to fit all the basics. The three of us chatted downstairs in the living room, which was littered with the trappings of triathletes: expensive-looking bikes, drink bottles, flippers, wetsuits drying on a clothes rack like strange abstract art. I wasn't sure how I was going to fit in there but the guys told me the room was mine if I wanted it.

Now, that room was crowded with debris from another life. Desperate to start ordering the chaos, I began putting clothes away into the new wardrobe. After hanging up my sweaters and new figure-hugging winter coat, I noticed I had brought my old jeans, which I'd not worn in nearly a year. Men's size 40 jeans. I held them up, amazed these giant swathes of denim had ever fit me. Why had I brought them with me? I sighed, threw the jeans down and brought my cold hands to my mouth, breathing on them, and saw the tan line and slight indentation around my ring finger. Too exhausted to continue unpacking or attempt to put the bed together on my own, I felt my body crumple like a piece of paper and fall onto the bare mattress on the floor. I curled up, fully clothed, too tired to cry again.

*

Having started my tenancy with a naked Ironman welcome, my first week in the share house was certainly interesting. I did my best to socialise with Ironman and Bomber, who were friendly enough but very much preoccupied with their own activities and lives. I'd never lived like this before; sharing a house with people I had no history with. Was I obligated to socialise or was I expected to stay out of their way? I didn't really have a clue.

My initiation into the house seemed complete when, late one night, I overheard what sounded like a porn film being made in the bedroom next to mine. I wondered if lying alone in bed, hearing the moans of strangers, would be the closest I would ever get to having sex again.

The fact it was winter, almost permanently dark and cold, suited me fine. It gave me an excuse to retreat. Most nights I got home from work and found the house empty anyway, so I would curl up on my mattress on the floor in my room, which was still a mess of boxes. The mornings were freezing. I would make tea and porridge, both so hot the kitchen window steamed up, to get warmth back into my depleted body, which to my perverse pleasure was looking even bonier these days. Meredith, who lived nearby, often offered to drop me in Parkville on her way to work, but otherwise I walked to the station and took the train to Flinders Street or Melbourne Central. At peak hour the trains were packed full, so I would just squeeze on, slide into an available sliver of space and stand, trying not to look at anyone, feeling the breath of strangers on my skin, wondering if anyone could tell what had happened to me by my still-marked ring finger, my sunken eyes, the emotional exhaustion plain on my face.

I'd emerge onto Swanston Street to the smell of coffee, traffic and fresh newspapers, and take a tram that trundled and creaked like a peddler's cart up to the university campus. My job was proving to be my saving grace, the one thing that was still holding my relatively new world in Melbourne together. I hadn't exactly made the news public there but the change to the nameplate on my door was a dead giveaway. I was surprised at how understanding and sympathetic my colleagues were. My originally part-time job had been made full-time – when I had broached the subject with my manager, a professor, explaining that now I was single and living alone a part-time income would not be sufficient, he had agreed straight away. 'Don't even think of looking elsewhere,' he said kindly. 'We'll make you full-time. That should be the least of your worries.'

One morning, after another lonely night and cramped commute, I arrived at work to find a patronising and emotionally blackmailing email from Glenn. We hadn't seen each other for weeks and in his emails he switched between saying he wanted me back and boasting about his fantastic new life. Why wouldn't he just leave me alone? Tears of frustration rolled down my face as I sat at my desk.

'Philippa? Are you all right?' It was the professor, standing in the doorway.

'Oh, yes, I'll be fine,' I squeaked, but for every word I spoke, a dozen tears spilled down my cheeks.

My boss comforted me, revealing that he too had been divorced and he completely understood the guilt, the grief and, of course, manipulative former spouses trying to claw back what they now realised they had lost. 'Be glad you didn't have children,' he offered as a bright side. 'That would have been even more painful.'

Much as I agreed with that, it was hard to imagine this situation being *more* painful. As well as the emotional heaviness, it actually physically hurt. Every morning when I woke up alone in the tangle of blankets on the mattress on the floor, the bed frame still resting against the wall like the skeleton of a whale, the memory of why I was there and everything that had happened would suddenly hit me. Fresh out of sleep, the sharpness of grief would flash like lightning through my chest. I didn't understand. I was genuinely relieved it was over, so I hadn't expected to feel this broken.

My boss pushed a box of tissues across the desk to me. 'Philippa, you'll get through this,' he said earnestly. 'You'll be happy again one day.'

I couldn't find the words or the strength to ask him . . . *How?* When everything I had ever known had fallen apart, how would I ever recover? Did I even deserve to be happy again? I was so weighed down with guilt that just getting through a single day was an achievement. I couldn't see any further than where I was.

But I did get through that day and enjoyed a cheap and delicious dinner at the Shanghai Dumpling House after work with Ashley and Meredith, who were both keen to hear how things were going in the share house, especially after the naked welcome. I shared my fears that I was utterly clueless when it came to this new life. I didn't know how share houses worked. I wanted the guys to like me and see me as a cool, fun housemate but felt I was failing miserably.

'Every share house is different, Phil,' Meredith reassured me. 'I've lived in places where the people were like family from day one, others where I barely saw or spoke to my housemates and it was just a place to crash. It all depends. You won't get to know these people overnight.'

I nodded. 'That's true. I've got to give it a bit more time, I guess.'

Meredith smiled, her face full of understanding. 'Seriously, they seem like decent guys. And living with people who call a spade a spade and give you your own space is just what you need right now.'

'Yeah. I know you're right. I just feel so lost.' I said. 'I really thought moving in there was the start of my new life and all this chaos would start sorting itself out, but it hasn't. If anything, life's even more of a mess.'

'Hon, that's totally understandable.' Ashley smiled sympathetically as the waitress darted in between us, taking away the empty plates. 'With everything that's happened, I don't think you can expect life to be normal for a while.'

Or ever, I thought. I didn't think it was normal to be twenty-five and getting divorced, a fact of my life that would never change, even with the passage of time.

Meredith and I caught the train home together and parted ways at the station. I wished I'd thought to bring some gloves. It felt like a layer of frost was slowly crusting on my hands. I kept them in my pockets as I walked the few blocks home, still needing to check the street names before turning down them.

I hated this time of day. Leaving work, staying in the city until tiredness wrapped itself around my bones and then finally going home in the dark to … what? I had no one to go home to any more. But I still had a home, I reminded myself. In fact, I had tried to establish my new presence in the house by brightening up the communal areas with some framed pictures, a few vases and bits of furniture to inject some familiarity into this strange life I was now living. I had been saddled with the bulk of the furniture, as Glenn had refused to take it, claiming there was no room in the soulless box in a Spencer Street high-rise he was now calling home. Glenn was sharing his new apartment with a thirty-something guy called Bert.

I'd giggled when he told me this. 'So you're going to be Ernie then?' Naturally, despite having told me thousands of jokes less funny than that over the years, Glenn had not been amused.

I turned my newly cut key in the front door, surprised to find the lights on and Bomber in the living room that adjoined the open-plan kitchen. He wasn't normally home this early.

'Hey, how are you?' I greeted him, wishing I'd put make-up on that day instead of deeming it a wasted effort because it would all be cried off before lunchtime.

'Yeah, good.' Bomber replied. He ran his hands through his hair. 'Uh, Phil, just a little thing. Can you keep your girly shit to a minimum down here, you know?' He gestured to my vases and ornaments, the framed photos of my family.

Great. Yet another thing I'd got wrong. I felt my blood pressure rise. What was the big deal? The house was mostly a dumping ground for Ironman and Bomber's bikes and triathlon gear, so what did it matter if I had a few personal things dotted about? It was as if they wanted no evidence of me living there at all. *Don't cry in front of him*, I thought as I felt the tears starting. 'I just wanted to make the place a bit nicer,' I said feebly, feeling like a child being told off.

'But this is a share house! You don't put family portraits in the living room.' Bomber rolled his eyes at the obviousness of it.

'I'm not being clueless on purpose, you know! I've never done this before. You could cut me a bit of slack,' I fired back, feeling defensive, no longer caring if I cried.

His expression softened. 'You'll be okay. Trust me, you'll get over it. You'll meet someone else.'

It amused me how that was everyone's token response whenever I was upset these days. I didn't want to just 'meet someone else'. In fact, another relationship was the last thing I wanted. I just wanted to stop feeling like shit every day, and to stop constantly putting my foot in it when it came to this new life where I didn't know any of the rules.

I started gathering up my 'girly shit'. Bomber wasn't the most sensitive guy in the world but even he could see my mask was slipping. He gently asked how I was settling in. 'Is there anything you need help with?'

My face lit up. 'Well, now that you mention it ...'

At least I would sleep in a bed that night.

The divorce diet

was surprised that, with my diet now built almost exclusively on peppermint chocolate, porridge, Chinatown dumplings and alcohol, I was continuing to drop the kilos. Every time I went clothes shopping I was a size smaller. Size 12 trousers I had bought at goal four months earlier were hanging off me. I got exclamations of disbelief and curious stares wherever I went.

'Phil! You're even skinnier than the last time we saw you!'

'I think you should stop now; there'll be nothing left of you soon!'

'You could do with putting on a few pounds, skinny!' (No one had ever said that to me in my life.)

'You look amazing! What on earth is your secret?'

Well, it's quite simple, I wanted to say. Basically, you spend nearly seven years of your life with someone you desperately loved at one point, but then slowly it dawns on you it isn't right and possibly never was. And while the thought of leaving breaks your heart, so does the thought of staying. Eventually things get so bad, leaving is your only option. So you pack what remains of your life into a few boxes and suitcases, and after that, live every day with shame, fear and guilt that eats you up from the inside. Shame because this is not what you wanted your life to be or who you thought you were. Fear that you are unlovable and branded for life because of this terrible mistake. Guilt that you took a vow and have had to break it to save yourself. Before you know it, the size 12 jeans are falling off you. Easy. You've never looked better.

I was so broken and in so much pain that I was questioning whether leaving had in fact been the right thing to do. I didn't appreciate that the end of my marriage was a loss and this was grief I was feeling. When you go through something like this, it takes time to adjust, to mourn the loss of the future you thought you were going to have and to reclaim your place in the world as an independent adult when you're so used to being part of a couple. In fact, I had never been an independent adult before. It was a lot to get used to.

One particular evening, I collapsed onto my train home, pulled out my book and tried to forget about life for half an hour. I was reading Paulo Coelho's masterpiece, *The Alchemist*, recommended to me by a blog reader. As the train left Parliament station, I came across a line in the book about how true love doesn't make you give up your dreams. If it does, Coelho says, it isn't true love. Those words made the chaos of peak hour around me stop still, like I'd entered a cave. I clutched the book to my chest and felt tears run down my face. If anyone was disturbed by the sight of me, they didn't show it. I knew then, beyond any doubt, that despite the pain I had done the right thing.

But every time I heard someone say to me, 'You're young, you'll meet someone else,' during those first few months, I wanted to cry with frustration. Didn't anyone understand? It was as if getting divorced at twenty-five was no big deal – I had enough youth on my side to be able to put the whole thing down to experience. Hardly anyone I knew had been in this situation. It wasn't like a usual break-up where you packed your things, left, and that was the end of it. I was legally bound to this man. It wasn't officially over. It felt like I was Glenn's property – in fact, he made a point of saying 'you're still my wife' to me on a number of occasions. Of course that was true, but I wanted all outward evidence of this obliterated. I changed my surname back to my maiden name, which was a hideous process, requiring endless official documents. When it was finally done, and I had replaced and destroyed anything that still had Glenn's surname on it, I vowed that, in the unlikely event I ever remarried, I would never change my name again. I was ready to find out who the hell Philippa Moore was.

*

As the weeks passed, I slowly acclimatised to the share house and felt less awkward around Ironman and Bomber, who were by far the most attractive men I had ever seen on a regular basis, but I was still very unused to some of their habits. For example, there was a white shoebox in the lounge room that housed Bomber's porn collection. I was shocked this was so out in the open but weirdly they didn't necessarily watch it to get off – they seemed to watch it for a laugh. Some nights I'd come in from work and the two of them would be in hysterics over some raunchy romp on the Panasonic screen. And Bomber's porn addiction didn't stop there. He thought it was the height of taste to plaster the kitchen cupboards with posters from his various girly magazines. The house was empty the night I got home and discovered this kitchen art montage. I cringed. Was this just part of life with two red-blooded Aussie men?

'Am I being a total square if I take them down?' I wondered aloud. I'd already been rapped over the knuckles a few times so far, but surely if I couldn't have my Wedgwood Bramble china, Bomber couldn't have his topless pictures! I know now that my time in that house would have been easier if I'd just had more of a sense of humour, but life felt very serious for me at that time and I felt that expecting me to turn a blind eye to posters of topless women in the kitchen was asking too much. There was no one around so I left a sticky note, glaringly yellow on the white cabinets, asking Bomber if he would kindly put these pictures in his room instead, and signed my name with a smiley face. I got changed, as I was having dinner at Meredith's, and headed out.

I got home late, wandered up the stairs and along the landing to my bedroom. Even without the hall light on, I noticed immediately that my bedroom door was covered in something. As I got closer I saw it was all the pictures that had previously adorned the kitchen cabinets, plus more. Every inch of the door was covered in bare breasts and firm buttocks and in the middle was the yellow sticky note. Bomber had drawn a line through 'Phil' and written 'Grandma'.

A decade on, this story makes me laugh, but at the time I was very embarrassed. I tore the pictures down angrily and threw open my bedroom door. I switched on the light and there was more porn on the bed – magazines opened to choice images Bomber presumably thought I would enjoy, mostly girl-on-girl action.

'Bomber!' I yelled. 'This is *not funny!*'

Bomber came out of his bedroom, topless, his six-pack visible in the dim light, and my heart leaped to my throat.

'Fucking hell, you've got to learn to have some fun,' he said.

I got my revenge a few nights later, when I decorated his bedroom door and bathroom mirror with a few examples of man-on-man action that I'd found among the flyers and pamphlets at a Smith Street cafe. Bomber barely raised an eyebrow, but perhaps it was reassuring to him that I did have a sense of humour, a spark of life lying dormant, somewhere.

Around this time Meredith and Justin encouraged me to sign up for a dating website, and even though it was a nice ego boost to start with, it became clear this wasn't how I wanted to meet someone. I got 'blown a kiss' by middle-aged men who had ignored the little section where I had clearly said no one over forty. I was even on the receiving end of some 'Why haven't you written back? Aren't I good enough for you?!' messages that terrified me and I had no idea how to respond to. If this was dating, I wasn't interested. I shut my profile down and went out for drinks with an attractive man I met on a training course at work; I thought the date went well but then I never heard from him again. I had no idea why until I was chatting to Bomber and Ironman a few nights later and told them the particulars. Apparently I had made a big rookie mistake.

'You don't tell a guy your life story the first time you meet him!' Bomber chastised. 'Of course you'll scare him off! It's a striptease. Reveal slowly!'

It all felt very hopeless. And it didn't help that I was still regularly hearing from Glenn. Good to see that my polite request for him not to contact me for a while had sunk in. Every time I heard from him I felt my body tense up with irritation. It had been nearly a month since I had last seen him, when I had dropped him off at the train station after we had finally cleared out the last of the things from our rented house in the outer north-west of the city. He had just looked at me, sitting in the passenger seat, not wanting to get out of the car until he saw the train approaching because it was cold, and said, 'I hope you'll be happy, Phil.'

I'd nodded, my eyes surely cried dry of tears, but no, there they were again. 'I think I will be,' I said quietly. 'I hope you'll be happy too.'

Glenn looked at me mournfully. 'I wish you could have been happy with me.'

I didn't know what to say. 'Well, I was once.' We let that hang in the air. 'It didn't have to be this way, Glenn.'

The train pulled up just as the words left my mouth. He got out of the car and walked away.

*

June and July had been very dark and emotionally intense months. I oscillated rapidly between being excited by the world of possibility that had opened for me with the end of my marriage and the growing readership of my blog, and, on other days, the failure of my impending divorce. The weight of it felt so heavy, as if those 28 kilograms I had worked so hard to lose had found their way back to me. It was exhausting. I had learned during my weight loss, however, to push through defeatist thoughts and stay positive, so I was doing my best to pump myself up and get through the days. I began to wonder whether everything had happened this way for a reason – that I discovered the real me as I'd shed the kilos over the past year, finding inner strength and courage to change something I wasn't happy about so I would later have the tools to deal with what I was going through now. Maybe the Universe did have my back after all.

Life continued to go on around me. It was a bit of a jolt back to reality that other people didn't stop getting married or engaged just because my marriage was over; that they didn't stop moving forward with their lives just because mine had stopped still. Ashley was now expecting her first child and was absolutely glowing with good health. We met for coffee one day and I gave her a bag filled with clothes – dresses and tops that had been part of my everyday wardrobe only a year earlier and that were still in good nick so I had put them aside to wear as maternity clothes one day. Now that pregnancy was certainly not going to happen for me in the near future, I wanted to pass them on. I was so happy for Ashley, yet also sad for myself. I had no idea what the future was going to hold for me now. But having spent the past seven years of my life planning a future that had now come to nothing, I was starting to think that was a good thing.

The blog continued to be a massive source of support for me, as were the real-life friendships I had made from it. I drew a lot of strength from that, and the validation I got from knowing my writing (as self-indulgent as some of it was at the time) was being read and appreciated by people all over the world started to help me believe I was not the most hopeless and unlovable human being on the planet. The kindness and understanding I got from everywhere at that time – from my family, my friends, my colleagues and my blog readers – was the glue that started putting my broken heart back together. Slowly, I started to feel alive and inspired again, and ideas began to come from everywhere. I began writing more and some days I felt dizzy with excitement about all the possibilities for my future. I clung to these hopeful feelings, knowing that soon the brighter days would outnumber the sad and lonely ones. The future could now be whatever I wanted. I reminded myself of that constantly. I was excited, despite everything. Who knew what I might be doing in a year's time – this time a year earlier, I'd thought I was happily married. A year could change everything.

*

One rule of share houses I was more than happy to obey was not stealing other people's food. Bomber's frozen pies, packet pastas and chicken nuggets held little appeal anyway, so when I found my shelf in the pantry bare one freezing late-August night, I drove to the supermarket in Ivanhoe, a few suburbs over. I had been running and was, despite the cold, wearing bike shorts and a hoodie, with my hair pulled into a tight ponytail and my face still streaked with sweat.

No sooner had I procured a basket and headed into the fresh produce section, than I saw Ironman, his trolley full, two boxes of condoms placed prominently on top of his loot.

'Glad I ran into you, Phil,' he said, grinning. 'I meant to remind you, it's your turn to buy toilet paper and dishwashing liquid and all that shit this month.'

'It's my turn already?' I asked warily, this being the first time any division of household expenses had come up.

Ironman shrugged. 'You got Rhino's room, you got his space on the roster.'

What roster? This was all news to me. 'Could we talk about this at home, do you think?' I was starving and not really in the mood.

Ironman headed to the checkout and I began grabbing vegetables indiscriminately, my stomach rumbling. I was breaking the cardinal rule of grocery shopping – never do it when you're hungry. Perhaps the same rule should apply to dating too.

As I made my way into the fruit section and snapped up a punnet of strawberries, I saw a handsome man in a suit standing by the bananas, gazing at me with a mixed look of recognition and awe. I smiled shyly and kept going. After resisting the urge to break into my selections while I shopped, I piled up my groceries at the checkout, packed them, paid for them and starting walking back out to the car park. It was freezing. The rigour of the run had worn off and I started to feel a little goosepimply in my tiny shorts.

'Excuse me?'

I looked around and into the smiling brown eyes of the handsome man who had clocked me earlier.

'I'm James,' he said. 'Have we met before?'

I smiled. 'Nice line.'

James looked adamant. 'No, really, you look so familiar! Do you go to my gym?'

'No, I don't go to any gym.' I started hopping subtly from one foot to another to keep warm.

He laughed. 'That's funny. You look like you work out.'

'Thank you, I think.' I grinned. 'I do work out. I've just been for a run. But I prefer running in the fresh air than on a machine staring into space.'

'I see.' He looked amused.

It went back and forth like this for a bit until James realised there wasn't any previous connection between us.

'So, you're clearly a gym-goer, then?' I asked, not bothering to hide my admiration of his impressive physique. He was about my height – but I'm quite tall, always the giant in the back row in school photos – and even under his expensive-looking grey suit, I could see there wasn't an ounce of fat on the guy. James admitted that yes, he was a gym junkie. He was there at 6 a.m. every week day and then headed straight to work. He was an employment lawyer with a large firm on Collins Street, often working crazy hours, and staying fit kept him sane. It turned out he was fanatical about what he put into his body too. He had a no-carb regime, especially after 5 p.m. Every meal he ate was strictly protein and vegetables. I noticed the contents of his shopping bags were mostly pouches of tuna, cartons of eggs and bags of spinach.

We ended up talking in the car park for the best part of half an hour, when I realised that my barbecue chicken would be cold and the tub of low-fat ice-cream I'd got for afterwards was probably turning into soup. But I was no longer interested in eating.

'I should get going,' I said. 'It's getting a bit cold out here.'

'Well, I would have come and talked to you inside, but I thought you were with that guy with all the condoms.'

'Ironman? God no, he's just my housemate!' I laughed.

'Can I give you my phone number?' James asked, smiling.

I smiled back, utterly thrilled that a man as attractive as James would be interested in me. This had been so unexpected. I typed his number into my phone.

'Why don't you send me a text so I have your number too?' he smiled.

I did just that. 'Your turn now.' I smiled and walked off, feeling light and giddy, knowing he was watching me walk away.

After a week of flirting via text, James asked me if I'd like to go out for dinner. I accepted, feeling somewhere in between thrilled and terrified. This was the first real date I'd ever been on in my entire life. I had never really considered the first time Glenn and I went out in public together a date; it had only been a movie and we'd been 'going out' for over a month by then. It had all been so long ago anyway, and to be honest, as a measure of self-preservation, I didn't think much about the happier times with him. My memories were now mostly the mistakes, the moments that had actually given me clues as to the future I would have with him, the moments I wished I had turned and run.

As I waited on the corner of Lygon and Grattan streets, I was very excited but also so nervous I was shaking. Was it too soon to be doing this? My marriage was barely cold in its grave. I hadn't told James anything about that yet and once I did he was bound to be turned off. Who would want to go out with someone who was getting divorced at twenty-five, public proof that they were a fuck-up? Maybe I should just cancel, save us both some heartache. I reached into my coat pocket to get my mobile to call James and feign a head-ache or a cold. But before I could unlock the screen, there he was.

'Well, this time we're going to eat food as opposed to just buy-ing it,' he said, smiling. There was a friendly hug and a kiss on the cheek and then he led me to a restaurant towards the city-end of Lygon Street. It was a bitterly cold night but the smells of garlic, pizza and charcoal grills imbued the frosty air with warmth.

James was the same friendly and easy company he had been in the supermarket car park a week earlier. We talked about life in Melbourne, our families, our jobs, and he asked me about Hobart. I slowly started to relax and tucked into my perfectly cooked por-terhouse steak, letting the pink juices stain the butter-coated pota-toes that James had requested not be served with his own steak. As we ate, he looked at me curiously over his glass of pinot noir with a soft smile on his face.

'So, tell me, Phil,' he said. 'How is it even possible that you're single?'

Ah, flattery. Despite my housemates' earlier warning to reveal slowly, I began to tell James the whole sorry tale. I figured if this was going to go anywhere he would have to know sooner or later. But I tried to reveal it without sounding damaged, bitter or, worst of all, pathetic, which was hard. The reality of it all was still sinking in. Also, a broken marriage was such a foreign concept to most peo-ple my age. Most of them had had far more diverse experiences and more freedom than me, but had not experienced something like like this. But this was all I had. This embarrassing, painful, seven-years-of-my-life-wasted mess. And the worst thing was that it wasn't even officially over yet. I was going to have to wait another year before I could file for divorce, before Glenn was well and truly out of my life. And even then, would he ever really go away? Whether I liked it or not, I was going to be an ex-wife, with an ex-husband. I hated the idea. I felt I might as well have a black line drawn around my ring finger, marking me as a failure, a warning to all who approached me to think twice.

But I couldn't think about that now. Here was James, an interesting and friendly man, wanting to know more about me, and he didn't seem to mind in the slightest that I was separated. In fact, his face was full of sympathy. If he was bothered by anything – my intake of carbs, or my revealing a whole month of dating's worth of relationship history in about twenty minutes – he didn't show it.

'I'm sorry,' I said. 'That was probably way too much to tell you on the first date.'

'Don't be sorry,' he said gently, wiping his mouth with his napkin. 'I'm glad you told me. It's filled in a few blanks, for sure.' He sipped some water. 'If you don't mind me asking, you're only separated, so is it really over? Or is there a chance —'

'No. It's over.'

The conversation thankfully moved on from my marital situation to travel, a subject I was passionate about despite never really having done any. James talked about his trips to Egypt and Greece, ancient civilisations that held more appeal for him than the theatres of New York City, the Dickensian alleyways of London or the canals of Amsterdam that I was interested in.

'I'd love to do more travelling,' James mused between sips of the ginger tea he had ordered for us rather than a calorific dessert, 'but I think I should probably buy a house instead. My sister's always telling me to settle down, get on the property ladder, get a bit of security, you know.'

I smiled and shrugged. 'I thought security was what I wanted too. It turned out it was the last thing I should have been concerned about. I've spent my entire adult life on the side of the fence that people always think is greener. It really isn't. If there's something you want to do with your life, you need to do it. Bricks and mortar and security can come later. A year ago, I felt like my life was so boring, that it was as good as over. And now, despite everything, I feel like the world is my oyster,' I concluded joyfully, looking over at James, who was looking back at me, his eyes smiling.

'I think you're quite incredible,' he said, his hand reaching over to mine, and I felt the colour rise in my cheeks and my stomach flip-flop, until I realised that he was only reaching for the teapot, which I obligingly pushed towards him.

'Incredible and resilient,' he added as he poured more tea, the warm sharpness of the fresh ginger steaming out of the cup. 'The world *is* your oyster. You go for it.' He smiled again and a lovely warm feeling flooded over me.

I like him, I thought.

After dinner, we walked back to James's car, which he had parked a few streets away, but our hands were inside our coat pockets, so there was no chance they would innocently brush. I wondered about chemistry. What did it feel like? When I looked at James I didn't feel gooey and tingly, despite him being very handsome, but I did feel happy. Happy that I was out on a date with someone, happy that I was, at least to the outside world, moving on. I knew that probably wasn't the same thing.

James drove me home and as the car got closer to the house the familiar nervousness started up again. What would happen? Was a kiss, or lack of, on a first date one of the most telling signs? James's various Celtic rings – he had about three – glinted in the darkness as he changed gears and turned down Station Street.

In the end, there was no kiss – not a romantic one anyway. Just a nice hug and a peck on the cheek, thanks for a lovely evening (me) and a promise to call (James) and then I went inside, not knowing whether I was relieved, disappointed or both. I'd had a lovely time but now he was gone I was having trouble even remembering what he looked like. And what was the point of 'dating' anyway? I'd already been married (legally I still was) and I wasn't even the slightest bit interested in finding another husband, which seemed to be the whole point of the exercise. 'The One' hadn't been the one at all. I just wanted some friendship, some companionship, maybe even some sex. I'd only ever been with Glenn. What on earth would it be like to be with someone else? I didn't allow myself to think about that too often for too long.

It was hard though. I was living with two Roman gods and Melbourne in general seemed to be absolutely chock-full of handsome men – on trams, in bars, in shops, walking past me in the street, all of whom I would appraise in my mind while running through the possibility of something happening between us. I was a walking contradiction – grief-stricken and heartbroken over my failed marriage, ashamed of what I thought it said about me, and yet full of energy and curiosity and urges I had never had the chance to let loose. I wanted to go absolutely wild, and to hell with the consequences. After the year I'd just had, surely I deserved a bit of fun?

Still high on the good time I'd had with James, I went into work the next day to find an email from Glenn waiting for me. It was as if he had suspected I was starting to move on, as the gist of it was that he still loved me and wanted to try again. *I'm ready to go to counselling now,* he wrote. *There's a lot I want to say and a lot I'm hoping for, but I'll save that for when we go to counselling.*

'When'?! I couldn't believe his arrogance. What the hell did he think I'd been doing for the past few months? Sitting around, pining for him? I had a bit of a cry, out of frustration more than anything, and after splashing some water on my face and making a strong coffee, I wrote a reply. I was furious and wanted to tell him where to go in the most animated language possible, but I knew any anger on my side would be punished, as it always had been. In exchange for a peaceful and straightforward divorce I was going to have to bite my tongue, which had been my fallback position during the entire marriage anyway. I would just have to keep being the bigger person until it was finally, legally, over.

I wrote that I was sorry to hear he was lonely and not coping well, but the time to go to counselling together was months ago, when I had first suggested it and there might have been a chance that things could have worked out. It was far too late for reconciliation now. I hit send and prepared for the worst.

Glenn's response came a few hours later, as I was leaving work for the day, and, as I suspected, it was a complete backtrack on his previous email. Did I think he was suggesting we get back together? He was sorry to disappoint me but it was obvious to him we had no future together and he was only suggesting counselling for 'closure' purposes.

Even though I'd predicted it, I was so angry my fists started shaking. Why did he keep doing this? God forbid he'd shown some vulnerability and it hadn't got him what he wanted. If he'd behaved with a bit more humility, perhaps I would have been less harsh and made an effort to at least try to be friends. I didn't want him to be lonely or unhappy. But right now, with the manipulative way he was acting and everything he had put me through the last few months, I wanted nothing to do with him.

My phone vibrated with a text message. It was from James, thanking me for a lovely time last night and expressing a wish to see me again. Soon. *I completely understand where you're at in your life right now*, he wrote, *and I hope you know there is no pressure from me at all. The fact you have come into my life is enough.* What followed was an invitation to see a movie the following Tuesday and then have dinner afterwards.

That text couldn't have come at a better moment. I smiled as I locked my office and headed towards the lifts. It was all about the future now, I told myself. *I'm moving on.* I repeated that mantra to myself all the way home.

The movie date went very well, the tofu and vegetable hotpot at Chocolate Buddha afterwards even more so, and finally, when James dropped me home later that night, he kissed me. It was strange, at least at first. I was so nervous. I'd had seven years of kissing the same person, so it took a while to get used to a different rhythm. I felt like I was learning everything again.

'Would you like to come in?' I asked as we broke away from each other, and James took my hand and kissed my fingers, one by one.

He smiled. 'Yeah, I could come in for a coffee.'

'Oh, sorry, I don't have any coffee,' I said, wondering to myself whether it would be permissible to sneak a few teaspoons out of Ironman's jar of Nescafé.

James looked amused. 'Oh, darling,' he said. 'It's just an expression.'

Sigh.

The next morning I felt like a new woman, and in the weeks that followed, I relaxed into James, into the sweet newness of him. I hadn't felt this way for years, possibly never. My heart leaped whenever my phone beeped with a message from him. We started spending most evenings together but James would still be up on the dot of six for the gym, even if we hadn't fallen asleep until after two. On Saturdays we'd walk around the CBD together, hand in hand like a seasoned couple, going into the health food shops on Elizabeth Street so James could stock up on his protein bars. I loved telling the story of how we met, or watching James tell it and glance over at me with warmth. We went for drives down to Williamstown, where we kissed on the pier and drank wine in bars at sunset. I even met his sister and brother-in-law over Greek salads in Prahran one afternoon. They were lovely and I felt positively dizzy at the thought of being accepted into the family fold so soon. James couldn't meet my family easily, of course, but my sister Claire came to Melbourne for a weekend visit and, feeling brave, I introduced her to James and they got along brilliantly straight away. He also met Meredith and Justin, who liked him very much and seemed to think things were moving in the right direction for me. I had to pinch myself that only three months ago I had still been clinging to the fraying sail of my marriage to Glenn. It honestly felt like another life, another person. Not this happy, confident cosmopolitan creature for whom Melbourne and new love were fitting like the perfectly measured bra.

'It feels so nice to be with someone again,' I confided happily to Meredith and Justin when the four of us were out for dinner and James had nipped to the bathroom.

'Someone, or him?' Justin asked perceptively.

I didn't answer.

*

James went to Sydney for three days on a business trip in September. The second night he was gone, I came home to find a vibrant bouquet of flowers on the doorstep. *Just because. Love, James*, read the card. I think I might have swooned. I got a bit of teasing from Bomber.

The third night, I went to a beautician Ironman recommended (he went to her himself) and embarked upon my very first Brazilian wax. Initially I was very embarrassed but five minutes in, I realised that embarrassment should have been the last thing on my mind. I gritted my teeth and swore, wondering how on earth I would ever cope with childbirth if I found a bit of waxing tough, but afterwards it felt incredibly smooth and sexy. I wondered what James would think once he was back.

The next night James flew back to Melbourne and he came over to see me straight away. And broke up with me.

It was the last thing I'd expected. I barely said anything as James spoke. Everything he said was more than reasonable so I found it hard to be angry or to disagree with him, but the way he talked about it was so emotionless, as if he was discussing a legal case. I couldn't believe this was the same man who had been brazen enough to approach me in a supermarket car park, who had sent me flowers 'just because' merely two days earlier. What had I done? Had I not kept in touch enough while he was away? Had I been too reticent about my feelings? Why had it all gone wrong … again?

James said he felt that we didn't really have a future together. He thought, given what I had gone through recently, I needed to figure out what I wanted. With all my passionate talk about going overseas (admittedly, I had mentioned it a lot) he knew it would be wrong to stop me going. He, however, wanted to start settling down, which of course was the last thing I wanted to do. But I desperately tried to get him to change his mind.

'I probably won't go away for another year,' I pleaded. 'It's a long way off. If we were still together by then, I thought we'd just figure something out.'

James shook his head sadly. 'We'd be in too deep by then, Phil. You know we would be. And I don't want to be the reason you don't follow your dreams. I think you need to be your own woman for a while,' he said, resigned.

The rest of the conversation was a blur. I eventually gave up on my 'Let's see where we are in a few months' line as it was obvious James had made his decision.

'I just can't be with someone when I know there's no future,' he explained. 'I know it sounds ruthless. I'm probably too logical for my own good.'

Logical? Cowardly more like it, I thought, sitting there feeling sad and confused. How did he know there was no future? He hadn't even

146

given it a chance. But something I was unable to acknowledge at the time was that this wasn't 'the One' or 'the real thing', certainly not at that early stage at least. It was a rebound relationship and, sadly, James had probably picked up on that and wisely decided to make a break for it before things got messy, because he wanted something more permanent. I don't blame him; he was a lovely person and deserved more than what I could offer at the time. But that didn't make it easier.

I walked James to the door, where he wrapped his arms around me. I buried my face in his shoulder, inhaling the scent of Qantas business class seats and freshly pressed linen, the only-just-getting-familiar smell of him creeping into the cracks of me. *Go, just go*, I thought.

After he left I wandered from room to room, all of them as empty as I felt inside. The biggest disappointment, to be honest, was that the pain of the Brazilian wax the night before had been a complete waste of time!

With the news of my marriage breakdown still recent, I now felt the double sting of humiliation when I had to start telling people it was now over with James too. I had even mentioned on my blog that there was a new man on the scene. What was I going to say now? I felt like an idiot even though I knew, grudgingly, James was right. We wanted different things and it was for the best, but I hadn't expected to be so sad about it. I had enjoyed being with someone again, feeling wanted, feeling happy. James had been filling a space that had been taken up all my adult life and now it was empty again I felt myself floundering. I just wanted to fill that empty space again as soon as possible.

The next week I went on a business trip to Canberra and got back to Melbourne late at night. The airport was packed and the line for a cab snaked back into the baggage claim area. I joined the queue and prepared for the wait, made far more pleasant and exciting by the person in front of me, who was one of the most attractive men I'd ever seen in real life. He looked like he'd walked off a magazine shoot – all tanned skin, perfect white teeth, sandy hair and an athlete's physique. We chatted for the half-hour it took to get to the front of the queue – to my delight, he could quote random *Simpsons* lines at will, as I could – but as we were going to opposite ends of the city it made no sense to share a cab and continue the conversation. He let me go ahead of him when we finally got to the front, and handed me his business card as we said goodbye, his fingertips brushing mine. 'Please call me,' he said.

That Friday night, I found myself opposite Cab Rank in a posh inner-city restaurant. Every eye was on us. I was in my new power dress, a 1950s-style shift clinging to every slender curve of the figure I was still getting used to, and he was the kind of man who drew attention immediately, whose charisma made the air change and whose gaze made your toes curl. His arm was in a sling – he had fractured it at a football game the day after we met – so his movements were limited, but despite this I was spellbound. Thirty-five years old, he was intelligent, educated, ambitious and well travelled, with an interesting career. He also wanted to know all about me, and having his undivided attention made me feel like the most fascinating and sexy woman in the world. We drank expensive wine and his eyes lingered on me as I spoke, our feet brushing slightly under the table, the air thick with tension.

I don't remember how or when it came up but eventually he casually mentioned he had a girlfriend back in Adelaide, where he was originally from. My blood ran cold, the physical equivalent of a power cut. *Right, so nothing can happen*, I thought as I drained my glass of shiraz. *He must just want to be friends.*

Of course, I was very naive. I was flattered – deliriously so – that a man as charismatic, powerful and good-looking as Cab Rank was even remotely interested in me. But the idea of being someone's bit on the side, when I'd just got out of an unhappy marriage, did not appeal either. I didn't want to be That Girl. I really didn't. But I was aching. The hurt inside me over what had happened with James, and with Glenn of course, was a gaping, weeping wound. I wanted to move on. I wanted to feel wanted. This man was driving me wild. I was a single woman. I was free. If anything happened, it was Cab Rank who should feel guilty ... surely?

While the atmosphere was tense with longing, it was easy to make conversation and overall we had a very fun evening. Cab Rank drove me home, one-handed, in his fancy car with plush leather seats. Before we took the turn on Hoddle Street to go north-east to my house, he asked me if I wanted to go back to his place instead. As tempted as I was, I said no. 'Break up with the girl in Adelaide first. Then we'll talk.'

A momentary look of disappointment washed over his face, which made my heart race even more. 'Are you sure?' he asked.

'Yes.' I said. 'I think so.'

After all, the guy's arm was in a sling. How good would it have been anyway?

I found out a few weeks later. Cab Rank went away on another business trip but called me nearly every day. I was very lonely so I took the calls and indulged in the harmless, I thought, flirty conversations. I wondered if he had time to call his girlfriend in Adelaide as well, as we were on the phone for hours at a time. Finally I had it out with him and said that if he wasn't going to end things with her first, there was little point in carrying on like this. He apologised, saying he hadn't meant to lead me on and he hoped we could be friends. When he flew back to Melbourne, he called and it was surprisingly nice to hear from him. He asked me to come around to his place in Elwood that Saturday for dinner and a movie. 'As friends,' he insisted.

Needless to day, I was still there on Sunday morning. We spent the whole day together, first in a cafe that overlooked the ocean, where we had lattes and blueberry muffins, then walking for hours along the beach, talking about life. Every time I looked at him I shivered all over, remembering his lips on my skin the night before. We bought ice-creams from a van near the lifesaving club that had a fierce handwritten sign in the window: 'We don't give change for parking. Don't even ask.' We both laughed at it. 'You'll put that in a book one day, I'm sure,' he remarked.

When we finally said goodbye late that afternoon, I drove home with the windows down, feeling the sun seep into my skin, singing along to U2 on the radio and watching the city shimmer like a mirage in the sunshine. I knew it wasn't the smartest thing I'd ever done. I still hadn't found what I was looking for. But I felt so alive.

*

Despite being terrified to be vulnerable in my personal life, I had no problems being so online. My blog was now password-protected – meaning if you wanted to read it, I had to email you a password – purely because I knew Glenn had been lurking on it, as he would often send emails mentioning things I had written about in my latest posts, including the fact I was now seeing other people. I didn't want him knowing what I was up to but I wanted to keep the blog going; it was Meredith who suggested I start a new blog with a password on it.

To my surprise and delight, many people wanted to read it. The day I announced I was 'going private', I got ninety emails within a few hours, from people all over the world, from Finland to South Africa. I was truly amazed that people so far away, people I'd never met, were interested in me and my life. They were all so kind, and it meant a great deal. Away from Glenn's prying eyes, I had been spilling all the details about my dating adventures and also about the joy as well as the heartbreak, confusion and inadequacy I felt as I adjusted to my new life. I had even written about the kicking incident back in May. Every time I logged in, it still felt like I was catching up with friends.

And so of course I wrote about what happened with Cab Rank, in detail I can't say I would use with complete strangers on the internet now. Having had nothing but support from my readers up to that point, I was taken aback when I got a handful of fairly scathing comments. I didn't understand. I was single – why was I the bad guy? I was, however, carrying on as though I were a character in a soap opera and I can see why that might have been irritating. Both online and off, I was completely high on the attention and thriving on the drama. It took my focus away from what was really bothering me. My moments of clarity were few.

I went round to my friend Ming-Zhu's a few nights later to help her with the catering she was doing for an indie film that was shooting the following day. We had been good friends at school, when we were both obsessed with literature, theatre, the need for expression and the need to escape. Only she had managed to escape at first, but having reconnected now I lived in Melbourne, we often hung out together after work in city bars, drinking wine and playing Scrabble, talking about life, art and our plans for both. Endlessly encouraging, her company was always uplifting and without fail she always made me think about something I'd never thought about before. As an actor she knew all about being in the moment and so, as we chopped and stirred that evening, I spilled all the beans on the Cab Rank saga. Unlike some friends I had at the time, Ming-Zhu neither egged me on, excited by the drama, nor judged me harshly for a lack of morals. She actually understood – I was lonely and, given everything I'd been through, I could hardly be begrudged a bit of fun. However, I was still doing something I knew was wrong and I had to own that.

'Honey, it's a free country,' Ming-Zhu reasoned. We had now finished cooking and were sitting with a glass of wine (essential for talks like this). 'If your conscience lets you sleep comfortably, then go for it. But I suspect there's more at play here than you just wanting some action. Am I right?'

Of course she was. The shame, the fear, the sadness – everything I'd been trying to forget about – was back with a vengeance and the familiar exhaustion was sinking into my bones. I had put that heavy load down once Cab Rank showed up and now, reluctantly, I had to pick it up again.

'I'm just so sick of hurting all the time,' I said. 'I feel like a failure, because it seems everyone I know is either getting engaged, moving in together, getting married, getting pregnant —'

'I'm not!' Ming-Zhu interrupted with a wry smile.

I conceded that, but she had to concede that she wasn't getting divorced either. 'I'm only twenty-five,' I sighed tearfully. 'I'm so angry at myself. I feel like I've done nothing with my life except waste time and fuck up. I just want to *live* for a while. And as for Cab Rank, I don't know … It was just nice to forget about all this shit for a while.' I reached for a tissue and wiped my eyes. Ming-Zhu squeezed my hand. 'I do feel bad though. I thought my standards were higher than that.'

Ming-Zhu looked at me thoughtfully. 'Philippa, we don't know what our standards are until we betray them,' she said.

It was the kindest thing that could have been said to me at that moment. This was a lesson I had clearly needed to learn. And I was beginning to realise I couldn't expect a cheering squad for everything I was doing either. Whether or not karma was going to kick me in the arse for this moment of weakness, who knew? But now I knew what my standards were, I couldn't betray them again.

Cab Rank stepped off the curb he came from and as he disappeared, that familiar aching emptiness returned. Why had something so bad for me felt so good?

There had to be other ways to feel good.

Cheaper than therapy

I was flicking through the *Herald Sun* as I waited for the coffee machine in the staff room to fill my mug with a much-needed black coffee. As I perused the sports pages I found an article on triathlons, specifically triathlons for beginners. There was going to be a series for beginners in Melbourne, starting in late spring and lasting all through the summer. The distances didn't look too scary. A 300 metre swim, 15 kilometre cycle, 3 kilometre run – none of those seemed impossible. It planted a seed in my head that grew over the rest of the day. I hadn't been all that focused on living the healthiest life lately, neither physically nor mentally. I was drinking more than I should and although I still ate fairly healthily, I often found I wasn't hungry at meal times, so I just wouldn't eat. I revelled in waking up with an empty flat stomach each day.

I was beginning to spiral into dangerous territory. My late nights were catching up with me as well. Something needed to change. I needed focus in my life again. I didn't want all my hard work in building up my fitness to go to waste. I needed to have some goals again, goals that didn't involve unavailable men.

So I ripped that triathlon article out of the paper, confident that mid-afternoon was a safe time to help myself to articles from the staffroom copy. When I got home I showed it to Ironman, who almost leaped off the coach with excitement.

'Yes! You've got to do it, Phil!' He was alive with enthusiasm. 'It's so much fun. You'll have the best time!' And, he said with a cheeky smile, triathletes tended to throw pretty great parties. I already knew that – he'd had one at our house a few weeks earlier and it had been like being at a *Sports Illustrated* model casting call.

Ironman told me about a coaching clinic he thought I should sign up for. He would help me with getting a bike and said I could borrow his flippers for swimming training. For a guy I hadn't had a lot in common with before now, he was being so kind and his enthusiasm was infectious. Before I knew it, I'd signed up for the first race at the end of November. But I was still terrified.

'I haven't done freestyle since primary school!' I moaned to Ironman. 'I don't have a bike! What the hell have I signed up for?'

He grinned. 'The ride of your life.'

The next six weeks flew by. I trained like a demon, with the same discipline I had displayed during my weight loss but had misplaced over the past six months. Every day I either went to the pool in Ivanhoe, or went for a ride or run on the bike track to Abbotsford Convent and back. I slowly built up my distances and stamina and was thrilled when I realised I had broken the 5 kilometre barrier with my running. How had this happened? A year earlier I had struggled to run for five minutes without collapsing. I still remembered every moment of that run, the ragged breathing, the burn in my thighs. At that time I thought I would never be a 'runner', one of those bouncy, shiny, ponytailed girls who glided along the pavement. Well, now here I was – a runner. Not particularly bouncy and shiny, but a runner all the same.

I bought a basic cheap bike from a shop on Heidelberg Road, with white trim, and I christened it Snowball. The first time I pedalled out, along the same route I ran to the Abbotsford Convent, I felt a freedom and a lightness that I hadn't felt for years. It was like I hadn't a care in the world. Cycling was hard though. I was surprised by how much it worked the thighs; I didn't remember this from pedalling around my neighbourhood and down to the jetty and back when I was a child. I was also pretty clueless about gears, and forced my way up the slight inclines of the bike track as it rose back to Fairfield, feeling the chains grinding, not sure if I was doing it right but not really minding as long as Snowball and I got home in one piece.

When it came to the swimming, I was far less confident. I was finding the 25 metre length of the Ivanhoe sports centre hard to negotiate without losing heart and breath, so was quite terrified about how I would cope with 300 metres in the choppy open waters of St Kilda beach. This was where the specialist clinic Ironman had recommended came in. I found myself down at the Elwood beach sports centre every Tuesday and Thursday after work to practise the finer points of triathlon – like what on earth 'transition' was, how to get off a bike gracefully and swim in the sea – with skilled coaches on hand. I struggled a lot initially but finally got the basics of it. The coaches were friendly and encouraging. I made a few new friends at the clinic, all of whom knew who Ironman was when I mentioned him, the same way the pizza place in Fairfield knew his regular order when he said his name. Ironman, as it turned out, had sprained his wrist falling off a bike, which would mean he was missing the first triathlon race of the season. He had been very down about it at first, but was now philosophical. Injury was part of life as a semi-professional athlete.

'I'll still be there to cheer you on,' he told me with a grin. 'You're not getting out of this!'

I had no intention of getting out of it. I was actually really enjoying myself. For someone who had never been particularly athletic, I was surprised by how passionate I was becoming about endurance sport. It gave me such a sense of achievement. It helped that my legs were slowly getting very toned too!

One Saturday, after I had completed early-morning ocean swim training with the squad in Elwood, I went back to the house, changed and headed back into the city to do some shopping. I was feeling tired, mostly from the early starts with triathlon training, then going to work all day and often training after work as well. I'd also felt on the brink of tears most of the morning. I hated to admit it, but I was lonely. My friends were lovely but they could only do so much. I just wanted someone to cuddle up with on the couch on a Saturday, someone to stroll hand in hand with on an afternoon walk, someone to wake up with every day, maybe even someone to make some plans with beyond the next weekend.

I want to say to the girl I was then, and to every single girl who feels a bit lonely: the absence of a romantic relationship in your life does not mean you're a failure. Use this time to learn to love yourself. Relish your own company. Find out what you love to do and spend your time doing that. Feed the passions in your life other than those between the sheets. Make time to nourish yourself. Nurture your confidence from within. You're wonderful. Don't look anywhere else for happiness. You already have it within you. And for God's sake, enjoy this time. It's freedom!

No, not listening, 2006 Phil? Okay. Let's keep going.

I walked into Myer on Bourke Street, browsed the beauty counters and sprayed myself with some expensive perfume, then walked over to the escalators. As I did, I noticed a gorgeous man with spiky blond hair and blue eyes coming the other way. He clocked me as well. There was a smile but I kept walking and stepped onto the escalator.

'Excuse me?'

I turned around and there was Spiky Blond. He was wearing some kind of uniform. He wasn't a police officer. Perhaps a paramedic?

'Do you know where the Ticketek office is?' he asked.

I replied that no, I didn't. But when the escalator stopped, eager to keep the conversation going, I walked over to the store directory, him following me, and helped him find which floor it was on. Spiky, who eventually introduced himself as Dan, seemed grateful. We got talking and he told me he was a nurse at the hospital on Royal Parade, which explained the uniform. His real passion was paediatrics and he was completing a specialist diploma to move into the Royal

Children's Hospital permanently. My heart melted a tiny bit when he told me all this. Everything about Dan seemed so gentle: his words, his gestures, his voice. And he was gorgeous.

We exchanged numbers and arranged to go out for coffee after he finished his shift a few days later. We met at Cafe Nova on Brunswick Street and he laughed when I ordered a skinny latte. 'You don't need to order "skinny" anything,' he teased. I was still getting used to people saying that to me, convinced they must mean someone else.

Dan was attentive, interesting and fun company, and made it very clear he wanted to see me again. Before I knew it, it seemed we were an item. I basked in the warm glow of his attention and the looks we got when we were out together. Not only was he incredibly handsome but he had the same rippled, gym-going body as James, which I now had the confidence to take full advantage of. They were heady days. There were dates to Thai cafes in Fitzroy, Sunday afternoons browsing the bookstore in Lygon Street, late movies at Crown Casino. When I wasn't working or training for the triathlon, I was with Dan. Life was a bit of a dream. But like with all dreams, I had to wake up eventually.

It was about a month later, the weekend before the triathlon. I flopped on my bed, waiting for Dan to call. He had texted on Thursday evening, saying he would call later to organise something for the weekend. It was now Sunday night and I still hadn't heard from him. I felt so stupid for deliberately clearing my weekend so I could jump whenever he crooked his finger. I hated that he worked unsociable hours and I was left waiting around all the time. He probably wouldn't even come to watch me in the triathlon at this rate.

Finally accepting that my stare did not have the power to make a phone ring, I went downstairs to see if I could join in on Ironman's usual pizza order. He was always keen to hear about my love life and of course it was all I wanted to talk about, so I spilled the latest with little encouragement.

'I don't get it!' I fumed. 'Why would you pursue someone, spend heaps of time with them and then just disappear?'

'Maybe he's met someone else,' Ironman mused.

'What?!' I was appalled, thinking of all the numbers I'd turned down and flirtations I hadn't indulged in over the past few weeks because I was supposedly Dan's girlfriend. We'd never actually talked about it, though he had said 'I love you' while leaving a voice-mail the week before. It must have accidentally slipped out, as he added, 'Oh, shit. I didn't mean to say that,' before hastily hanging up. I hadn't known what to make of that. He certainly hadn't brought it up.

Ironman reached for another slice of pizza. 'Or maybe he's got back together with that ex you said he kept talking about. You've only been seeing the guy for a month or so, it's not like you got married.' He paused and then looked at me. 'Did you?' he teased.

I pulled a face at him. 'No!'

Now that I thought about it, things had become strange with Dan lately. In the early days I used to hear from him all the time, but now the gap was longer between texts or phone calls. He had been three hours late for our last date and hadn't seemed that sorry about it. Any suggestions he meet any of my friends were met with excuses, and he always stayed at my place; I had never been to his. Ironman was right. There had to be someone else. Either that or

160

Dan had lost interest and was hoping that by being thoughtless and distant, I would break it off with him. I didn't know which was worse. I remembered a comment left on my blog at the height of the Cab Rank drama: 'How would you feel if you were the girlfriend?' Perhaps I was getting exactly what I deserved.

Ironman thought I should just forget about him. 'Concentrate on the triathlon instead. Come on, you've worked so hard. That's the thing to be focusing on.'

I nodded. 'You're right. I haven't worked this hard to throw it away for some arsehole who can't be bothered.'

I wish I believed it. I still felt having no man in my life and my impending divorce meant that anything else I had to show for myself didn't count for much. I put my head in my hands. I felt so pathetic. So much for being a strong, independent woman then. No one had told me being single would be this hard.

*

The day of the triathlon dawned and Ironman knocked on my door at five. He put on some house music to pump up the atmosphere downstairs. 'Woo hoo!' he hooted, pouring coffee and grinding his hips to the music as if he was in a nightclub. I was so nervous I could barely eat anything, but I somehow managed a Power Bar. We loaded up the car with my bike and kit bag, which I checked the contents of about a thousand times, and then we drove to St Kilda. Hoddle Street at six in the morning was a revelation. The normally choked street unfolded as smooth as silk and we were at the Fitzroy Street turnoff in about ten minutes. The city was so still and peaceful.

Ironman and I approached the tent, where the coaches from the beginners clinic gave me words of encouragement, helped me put the stickers on my bike and helmet, and wrote my competitor number in thick black marker on my right thigh and upper arm. I went to the transition area – where your bike, running shoes and other gear you need for the next stage of the race are kept – to rack Snowball and set up my kit, grease my shoes with vaseline and talcum powder, place my helmet and sunglasses in an open position so I could put them on quickly. It was an operation of military precision. I'd lost Ironman at this stage, as he had been swept up in his throng of admirers, so I went down to the water and ducked in to warm up. It was absolutely freezing and I leaped out as quickly as I'd got in and then waited on the shore for my wave to start. Suddenly my nervousness vanished. I felt surprisingly calm. Finally the horn blasted and the race began.

The swim was the hardest part, as I'd expected. I reverted to breaststroke when I felt fatigued, which was almost immediately. I freaked out a little when I felt other legs kicking next to mine and felt someone else's hands near my head as we swam around the cans and then back towards the shore. As I ran out of the water I saw Ironman at the front of the cheering crowd, waving and cheering, 'Go, Phil!'

My heart swelled with gratitude for him. I ran from the beach back to transition, where I strapped on my helmet, slid my cold feet into my greased shoes and took off on Snowball down Beach Road. It took a long time to feel comfortable in the ride because my feet were numb and I didn't feel in control enough to go all out. The wheels and pedals spun wildly as I commenced the descent towards

Luna Park, my fingers clutching the brakes most of the way down. The sun had fully risen and the sky was clear.

I went back into transition to rack Snowball, dump my helmet and head out for the run. It was only short, from Catani Gardens down to Luna Park and back, but the tightness in my thighs from the furious bike ride made it more of a challenge. I tried to concentrate on my surroundings. I had worked hard for this, albeit as a distraction from the dramas in my life. I wanted to enjoy it. I watched the early-morning walkers with their dogs on the sparkling white sands of the beach, the rickety rollercoaster tracks of Luna Park glittering in the sun, the St Kilda cafes slowly opening for breakfast. Finally I saw the sign that told me I only had 400 metres to go and I sprinted with every ounce of strength I had left. The anger and frustration I felt at all of them – Glenn, James, Cab Rank, Dan – burned inside me and made my legs move even faster. I ran and ran, overtaking about five people as the dust gathered behind me and the finish line came into sight. I crossed the line, had my electronic timing chip cut off, and then there I was. I had completed a physical feat that only a year ago would have been completely beyond me. I looked down at the black number on my looking-rather-muscly right thigh and remembered struggling to do up size 18 jeans in that Kmart changing room, only last year. In that moment, I allowed myself to feel nothing but pride. I had come such a long way.

*

After the wonderful high of the triathlon, I toppled off it to a new low. My relationship with Dan, if you could call it that, really hit the skids and eventually he just disappeared. I didn't understand why this kept happening. It wasn't that I wanted anything serious, as many people around me assumed. I was simply tired of letting my guard down and getting involved with someone, and then being either dumped or left hanging. And with every relationship that petered out, I was reminded of the great big failure constantly hanging over me. My broken marriage was the first thing I thought about every morning when I woke up and the last thing I thought about before I went to sleep. The grief wasn't as sharp as it had been in July, but it was still a jolt back to reality where I wasn't the sexy star of Melbourne's hottest soap opera, *The Secret Life of Phil*, after all, just a soon-to-be-divorced, needy twenty-something whose life was a mess. I just wanted the hurt to stop. I didn't understand why I was still so broken – I hadn't seen Glenn for months and had barely heard from him. I certainly didn't miss him. I was just tired of feeling sad all the time. I didn't comfort-eat any more but what I'd replaced that habit with was just as unhealthy. I could see myself repeating certain patterns with the men I dated that had flourished in my broken marriage: submission, passiveness, doing whatever it took to keep other people happy and swallowing all my hurt and anger, as if they had no right to be expressed.

Several friends were worried about me and encouraged me to see a counsellor again. I had no interest in going to see Iris, who had been as useful as a fishing rod in a desert, but one Saturday I dragged myself to a yoga class, my first in months, hoping that being inverted in downward dog for a while might give me some perspective. Immediately following yoga was a meditation class. The first class was free and I had nowhere else to be. I figured my mind could do with learning how to be quiet.

My manic mind found meditation very difficult indeed but I liked Jules, the teacher, and chatted to her afterwards. Jules took one look at me and said, 'Meditation is a very worthwhile skill to learn, especially if you're going through a hard time.' It turned out Jules was also a counsellor based not far from me. She said I was welcome to pay her a visit to see if she could help me.

It took me a few more nights of angst before I finally snapped and decided I didn't want to keep living this way. I wanted to be in control of my feelings and thoughts rather than be constantly held ransom to them. I had felt so proud of myself six months ago, when I got to goal, but now it seemed I had reverted to my old critical thinking, always feeling like I wasn't good enough. I wanted to know why I behaved the way I did, why I thought what I thought and how I might be able to fix the things that were holding me back. I had come a bloody long way on my own in the past year but if I needed help now, I was ready for help. I took a deep breath and rang Jules, who could fit me in the next day.

Although only a few minutes' walk from the noisy traffic of Heidelberg Road, Jules's cottage exuded calm. It was as if I were crossing a border. She welcomed me and led me into her consulting room, another oasis of calm with pure-white walls, minimal furniture, a single candle burning. Jules poured tea from a cast-iron teapot, and the aroma of steamed rice filled the air. In that peaceful room, I felt safe, and slowly unravelled. I said things I had never said out loud before, things I hadn't even fully gone over in my own head. It spilled out of me. I thought it would never stop. After I stopped speaking, Jules looked at me with warmth and empathy.

'Philippa, there are two main things I've drawn from what you've said to me. The first is that you are *allowed* to feel angry. You have the right to that feeling, and also the right to express it.'

That was something new. Anger and I had never been good together. I had been a placid, affectionate child; the terrible twos seemed to have passed me by, Mum was fond of saying. The few times I had ever got angry as a child I had been shot down so quickly I had been too terrified to ever do it again. Expressing any negative feeling, however justified, made other people upset and uncomfortable and, in my desire to be a 'good' person, I didn't want to do that. Therefore if I ever did feel angry I had to keep it to myself. Likewise, if people were nasty to me, rejected me or teased me, I couldn't get angry back at them, because that would make it worse. I simply had to endure it. This was not a good place to enter adolescence from. My all-girls school became a battleground. I was an easy target because I never fought back. I didn't know how.

Jules listened politely to my protests and then continued. 'But the second thing is that you need to work on *how* you express yourself. You internalise a lot. You need to get better at communicating with people and not being afraid to tell them what you need from them. But that's something we can work on together.'

I left Jules's house feeling a lot calmer than I had in a long time, feeling more like myself, and feeling like someone finally understood. It was the beginning of the healing.

The travel bug

'If adventures do not befall a young lady in her own village, she must seek them abroad.'

– JANE AUSTEN, *NORTHANGER ABBEY*

I started seeing Jules every Monday evening, when I would shed a few tears over situations where I had felt rejected or vulnerable, and we would gently unravel my feelings to get to their roots. It became clear that my inability to voice hurt, disappointment or anger with anyone for fear of losing them was slowly poisoning me. After everything that had happened with Glenn, I still felt unable to put myself and my needs first.

I came away from every session feeling enlightened but still incredibly low. There was always something to work on, more feelings to excavate and explore. In the meantime, I enjoyed going out on the town with my girlfriends, and revelled in whatever attention I got, but then felt deflated if I went home alone, or without a few phone numbers at the very least. I didn't know how to make myself feel better so I gave in to this needy behaviour, wanting other people to validate me, and yet remained puzzled as to why it turned any decent man off.

Another thing that counselling had uncovered for me was that I was tired of feeling afraid all the time. It had kept me stuck – to places, to relationships, in bad patterns. I talked to Jules about how I longed to go travelling, to live and work in London, but I was scared and didn't know why when this was all I had ever really wanted to do. I couldn't remember a time when I didn't want to travel. I think it coincided with my discovery of books at about age four, when my father would take me and my sisters on weekly excursions to the state library and I would pore over picture books about life in other countries. There was a series I particularly loved that followed a schoolboy or schoolgirl around, capturing their daily life in words and pictures. I was fascinated by these books about China and Japan, full of photos of schoolgirls barely older than I was, their classrooms with blackboards on which unfamiliar characters were written neatly in chalk, parks they played in, which had different flowers and trees, and their meals of exotic noodles, not the meat and three veg I was accustomed to. While my life in Tasmania was comforting, familiar and had ample to occupy me as a child, I yearned for adventures, to see all the things I'd only ever read about or seen in movies or on television. I had planned to travel while I was at university or once I completed my degree, like so many other people my age were doing. But all those plans went out the window once I met Glenn. I became very afraid of my big dream. Afraid of travelling alone, afraid of missing him if I left him behind, afraid that he'd leave me if I went without him. It never occurred to me that the thing to be truly afraid of was letting my dreams slip away. The weekend we moved into our brand-new house in 2004, after all the boxes and furniture had been brought in, I left them where they were and collapsed in a heap. All I did for the rest of that weekend was sit and read Lonely Planet guidebooks. I had everything I was supposed to want, except what I wanted most of all.

Spending Christmas 2005 in New Zealand gave me a taste for what else was possible. The day before that horrible night in May, I had booked flights to Christchurch for Glenn and me for October, a trip we still ended up taking, but separately. Glenn insisted on still going, as it technically had been his birthday present. A friend who worked for Jetstar kindly separated the tickets so we didn't have to sit together; we had a frosty reunion at the baggage carousel in Christchurch and then I thankfully didn't see him again. I stayed with a lovely blogging friend, Katie, and had a wonderful few days seeing all the city had to offer.

My time in Christchurch was up all too quickly and rather than return to Melbourne on the same flight as Glenn, I hopped on a plane to Auckland instead to visit my blogging friends there for a week. Emily and Jonny hosted me but I was truly honoured that other bloggers came up from Rotorua and Wellington to see me too. My time with Emily and Jonny was the most soothing balm for the soul I could have asked for at that time. They are such beautiful, genuine people, and I have never forgotten the kindness and generous hospitality they showed me.

While my travels in New Zealand only intensified my desire to see more of the world, when I got back from the trip in October 2006, life became busy with triathlon training and my new romance with Dan, so my dream was conveniently shelved once more. But then I began counselling and my dream started piping up again, falling into every conversation. My yearning for adventure would need to be satisfied sooner or later. I had been hitting the snooze button for a long time.

*

I went down to Hobart for Christmas where, despite having a mostly lovely time with my family, things were sometimes a little difficult and disappointing too. While I found it very hard to voice my needs in intimate relationships, I was more assertive with my family than I used to be and that didn't always go down well. In fact, it just seemed to make everyone sad about how much I had 'changed'. I was upset because I felt they weren't cutting me much slack, and they were upset because they apparently missed the old Phil. *Why would anyone miss her?* I thought angrily. Old Phil was a doormat and wouldn't say boo to a goose. I was glad I wasn't her any more.

When you go through a dramatic life change, people don't always react in the ways you think or hope they will. I can see, a decade on, that witnessing me change so dramatically in such a small space of time must have been incredibly hard for my family. But at the time, their various reactions seemed to validate my deepest fears – I was showing people the real me and they didn't like it.

The day after Boxing Day, I met up with my cousin Sally, who I hadn't seen for a few years. We met for coffee at Pane Cucina in Elizabeth Street, sipped lattes and caught up on each other's lives. She and her partner had spent nearly two years living in London but had returned to live in Sydney a few months earlier. She regaled me with tales of living in Putney, working in the city, the tubes, the markets, the museums, flitting off to Paris or Rome for a weekend. I felt my heart dance a little as she spoke. I wanted that life too, so very much.

As we hadn't seen each other since 2004, Sally was quite stunned by the physical change in me. She, on the other hand, was the same leggy, gorgeous blonde she had always been and to my great pleasure we actually looked like we were related now! She had heard on the family grapevine that Glenn and I were no longer together but she didn't know the particulars of what exactly had led to the split. As if my skinny latte were a truth serum, I told Sally everything. She looked horrified. But once I finished talking, she grinned and the look in her eyes was one of great respect.

'Well done for getting out of that,' she said. 'You deserve so much better.'

Sally wanted to know what I was going to do next and I told her I wanted to do exactly what she had done – live in London, meet new people, travel, have adventures – but I was terrified. She looked at me with surprise.

'Phil, after what you just told me, why are you so afraid of going overseas? It would be so easy in comparison.'

'But I'd be giving up so much,' I said. 'I don't know where to start. What if it's a disaster?'

'After the year you've had? I think you can survive anything.'

*

I arrived back in Melbourne with a renewed sense of vigour. For the next few weeks I pored over travel brochures collected from the travel agency on the university campus, looked at satellite maps of London streets, wondering where I might live, and looked into visas. It was a bit mind-boggling but I was so excited. What on earth had I been waiting for? If I didn't do it now I probably never would. I finally had no one and nothing to hold me back. Yes, it would be hard, but that was kind of the point – if it were easy everyone would be doing it. If leaving turned out to be the wrong thing, then I could live with that – and I could always come back. I couldn't live with any more wasted time and broken dreams.

A new era had dawned at the Fairfield house with the arrival of 2007: Bomber had moved out with his girlfriend, Ironman went up the ladder into the more spacious bedroom with ensuite, and Ironman's old room was taken by his wonderful friend from university, Louise, whose company I thoroughly enjoyed. We would often sit with a glass of wine in the evenings or go for a run together. One night as I was leaving yoga class, Louise texted to say she was cooking dinner. There seemed now to be a real sense of community and family in the share house, not just three people crashing in the same space.

However, despite this, Melbourne was becoming a claustrophobic and somewhat lonely and awkward place to be for me, and I was becoming more and more convinced that I didn't want to stay. The summer heat, combined with the emotionally exhausting work I was doing with Jules, added to the heaviness.

I hadn't seen Glenn for months but he had sent an email at Christmas, obviously feeling reflective with the impending end of the year and all that had happened over the course of it. He said he was sorry he had let me down and that he hadn't been the man I needed him to be. I had responded, thinking that maybe things could improve between us now, though I still had no desire to see or hear from him regularly. But the humility in that email disappeared very quickly and he continued to try to have the upper hand. He never asked about me and what I was up to, because, of course, that wasn't the point.

Meredith had also started acting strangely. The regular lifts she used to offer to work had dropped off and when I did see her, there was a coolness, as if she was longing to give me a good telling off. There had been one or two occasions, especially in the aftermath of being dumped by Dan, when I'd been a bit oblivious and not the most thoughtful friend in the world, but I had apologised unreservedly for upsetting her and thought we had moved on. I was too emotionally drained and afraid to find out what I'd done this time. Going out with Ashley without asking her along too? Giving Justin a hug that lingered a little too long? Talking to a guy on the train while she was with me? It was those sorts of things that Meredith had been getting shitty with me about lately. She seemed determined to take everything I did personally, which just wore me out.

My friendship with Meredith, as young as it was, had always been quite intense and, looking back, we were both very needy in different ways. I needed reassurance and support during a difficult time in my life, and I think she needed to be needed, especially by someone she looked up to. In the immediate aftermath of my separation and move to Fairfield, I had seen Meredith nearly every day for a while. Seeing me so raw and fragile after everything that had happened with Glenn, Meredith offered herself as a shoulder to cry on and always seemed very concerned about my wellbeing. I was so grateful for her presence in my life at that time. But now, six months later, things were very different. I was starting to stand on my own two feet again and didn't feel as dependent on my friends any more. I began to notice how possessive Meredith was and, far from making me want to spend time with her, it made me feel suffocated. I didn't feel good about myself when I was around her any more. Jules encouraged me to set some healthy boundaries, assuring me that it wasn't my job to take care of Meredith; she was an adult and responsible for her own feelings after all. But having had such an intense friendship so far, pulling away, even slightly, even with the kindest of intentions, was never going to go down well.

I can see a lot of friendships in this period of my life followed a similar pattern – people who were the best friends I could ask for in times of trouble then got upset or distant with me when I recovered and was less dependent on them. At the time, however, especially with Meredith, I didn't have the self-awareness to realise this was what was happening. I just thought that people who claimed to care for me and who had seen me through some hard times would be pleased I was beginning to come out the other side. I have since observed that it's a change for the better, rather than a downward spiral, that reveals who your true friends are, and sometimes you don't have as many of them as you think.

I realise I wasn't the easiest person to be around at that time either. I was a bit wrapped up in myself and needed people to talk to and cry to. Mad with grief and heartbreak, delirious on attention and validation, my confidence sky-high one minute and non-existent the next, I needed patience, reassurance, friendly ears and caring people who were not going to take anything I did or said that seriously. It did seem that life had gone from one extreme to the other – having lived my entire life up until now always worrying about what other people thought and wanted, I was now entirely focused on myself, which made me a bit oblivious to other people's needs, I'm sad to say. I think some people mistook my sudden narrow focus on my healing and getting my life together as a sign I didn't need or care about them any more, which of course was not the case at all, but I can see why they might have felt that way. Most people in my life were kind enough to realise it wasn't personal, but others made it clear they were hurt and disappointed, which I didn't know how to deal with. I had had a massive life upheaval and was coping as best as I could. Should I have tried harder to keep other people happy? I don't know. But whatever crimes I committed at this time, I was not expecting the punishment I eventually got.

It felt like everything had changed. Ashley had given birth to a baby girl just before New Year and had been sucked into the vortex of motherhood and all its trappings. While I still saw her, it naturally wasn't as often. Other previously close blogging friends like Gillian had become rather cool and distant, as Meredith was. Remembering the comments they left on blog posts I wrote at the time, their affection for me had clearly waned, and perhaps they were hoping I would eventually topple off the pedestal they had put me on in the first place. On the other hand, another blogging friend, Angela, who I'd become quite close to over the past few months, had made noises about wanting to visit when I moved to London – in fact, she insisted on booking flights barely a few weeks after I booked my own.

'I'll come and stay with you and we'll go off around Europe together. It will be fantastic!' she gushed.

While I loved the idea of a friend visiting, surely it would make more sense for her to wait until I'd moved there? It was obvious she wanted to be a part of my big adventure, even though it hadn't yet started.

'I have no idea where I'll be living or what I'll be doing,' I said carefully, knowing if I was too blunt she would get upset. 'You can book flights if you want but I hope you understand that I can't guarantee anything when I haven't even moved there yet.'

Angela brushed off my concerns, saying of course she understood that, and continued making her plans in earnest. I tried not to worry. I was trying to put myself first instead of worrying all the time about what other people thought. But that was proving to be easier said than done.

*

January was also going to hold what would have been my fifth wedding anniversary. I had already decided that I would escape Melbourne for the weekend. This was not going to be the weekend of mourning what might have been; this was going to be the weekend that something else happened. On a whim, I emailed Mary in Sydney.

If I came to Sydney next weekend, could we hang out?

Hell yes! came Mary's almost instant response. *You can stay with us if you like. Assuming of course that you're not a psycho.*

Or that you aren't, I replied.

Ok, you're staying with us, but we both reserve the right to pull out if we decide the other is a psycho.

It was just what I needed. I was desperate to get away. But yet again, some of my friends seemed mad that I was doing something without them. The day I left, as Meredith dropped me off at work for the first time in a while, she told me she was feeling very rejected by me of late. I didn't know what to say – 'I'm sorry you feel that way, but this isn't about you'? I think I did say words to that effect, as gently as I could, but I'm not sure. I know I didn't have the guts to tell her the truth. Our friendship couldn't handle conflict as we were both clearly terrified of it. I was starting to feel very alone, and that everything was changing.

Sydney, on the other hand, was pure fun, as were Mary and her partner, Daniel. I caught a taxi to their house in Newtown, a rambling semi-detached Victorian terrace in a street lined with frangipani trees. I was welcomed with hugs, pizza and beer. Mary was as warm, straightforward and funny in person as she was on her blog. She was passionate about yoga and dragged me along to her usual 7.30 class the next morning, which was amazing – I felt refreshed, cleansed, purged of my sadness. I felt empty but in a good way: emptied of all the sad things, the things that had been weighing me down, and ready to be filled again. I revelled in the clouds of smoky incense, the spongy purple yoga mats, the altar adorned with flowers and candles, the entire class chorusing, 'Om.' It was beautiful and magical.

After yoga and breakfast, we started preparations for a barbecue Mary and Daniel were holding in my honour in their surprisingly roomy backyard, which had plenty of drooping gum trees for shade from the frighteningly hot sun. Most of the guests were also bloggers, all of them regular readers and commenters on my blog. It was like walking onto the set of a favourite TV show, where I was a character as well. I also finally met M, who waltzed in just as the first sausages were put on the barbecue. She was as lovely in person as I'd always imagined she would be.

The Sydney blogging crowd were a merry lot. The backyard was alive with laughter, conversations, sizzling meat, ice cracking in the eskys. I looked around and knew that this was the perfect way to be spending the day – with new friends, making new memories. The hours melted like the ice keeping the drinks cool; there was music when Daniel and some of his friends brought out their guitars and harmonicas; the sun eventually dissolved into a molten-black night as some guests departed and new ones arrived. There was a never-ending circle of people to meet. I had to admit that spending a whole Saturday drinking and eating was not how I imagined hanging out with a bunch of weight-watching bloggers, but I loved every minute of it. I felt enclosed in a circle of support. Most people there knew what the day had been in my old life.

It surprised me how little I had thought of Glenn, and how faded my memories of our wedding day were. I only remembered fragments now: the faded carpet of the church aisle, the happiness on his face as I walked down the aisle towards him, the confidence in his voice as he said his vows, the sweet smell of the flowers I carried. But I still couldn't listen to the first song we had danced to without crying. Crying for what, I didn't know. The closest I could come to explaining the feeling was that someone had died. And it wasn't Glenn I was mourning. I still didn't know what it was I had lost; I just knew I would never be able to get it back.

It was about 2 a.m. when they finally kicked out the last stragglers and we headed upstairs to bed. 'You did good today, sister,'

Mary said gently. 'This day means something else now.'

Everything meant something else now.

*

I returned from Sydney feeling happy and light, a diamond bar in my newly pierced navel (Mary convinced me to do it!), completely ready for the next adventure. I finally bit the bullet and sent off my UK visa application. It could take a few months to come through so I figured I would book the flights once I had it. I continued to feel restless in Melbourne, filling my days with work and my nights with yoga classes when I could afford them, or going out for drinks with Ironman and Louise, or people from work I was friendly with.

I met a 22-year-old blond surfer on one of these nights, who I'll call Kurt, as he was quite similar in looks to the rather more famous Kurt Cobain. Kurt was quite smitten and wanted to see me again. With nothing else to do, I agreed. Kurt reminded me of a puppy dog – sweet, loyal, and very willing to be put on a lead. We arranged to meet for cold beers at the Espy in St Kilda and I could have sworn his tongue was hanging out of his mouth as he watched me talk. But I didn't do all the talking. It turned out Kurt was a bit of a revhead and currently had about $20,000 in unpaid speeding fines. He admitted to having once driven from Port Douglas to Melbourne in twenty-four hours. There had been speed involved, and not just the kind that's measured in kilometres. So that rather major incident and about two dozen others had resulted in his losing his licence about four times and receiving fines he had never paid, and now there was a warrant for his arrest. Somehow he thought it was magically going to go away. He rode waves on the weekends on the

Great Ocean Road, but that was all coming to an end soon because he had lost his licence again.

In ordinary circumstances, there would have been no second date for Kurt but my plans to travel and leave Australia indefinitely were now in motion and I'd given up expecting anything from men. No commitment, no long-term future, just a bit of fun with no strings attached. I figured a 22-year-old guy like him would feel the same way but, to my greatest surprise, he had very different ideas. He told me how much he wished he could join me on my overseas adventure, but with the unpaid speeding fines and a warrant for his arrest he would never be issued with a passport. I was deeply relieved that that was the case.

Eventually, after one of his housemates telling me that they had never seen Kurt so smitten with a girl, I decided the kindest thing, for all concerned, was to be brutally honest and tell him I would soon be leaving Australia, I wasn't sure when or if I'd be coming back, and I hadn't been after anything serious.

Kurt cried when I broke this news to him.

'But if you're not going for a few months, why do we have to break up now? Can't we just see if we're still together and sort it out then?' he sniffed.

This sounded very familiar. My mind drifted back to six months earlier and I realised I had asked James the same thing. If anything, it was worse being on the other end of the conversation. Is this how James had felt, watching me get teary and effectively bargain with him? I was also horrified to realise how much Kurt reminded me of Glenn when we had first met. Glenn, then the same age as Kurt was now, had also been emotional and immature, saying things to me that, at age eighteen, made me swoon and think him romantic but that now made me cringe.

Within ten minutes of leaving Kurt's house, I recieved an 'I miss you' text. The next night he called. And the next. Eventually, I stopped picking up the phone. Then he started sending emails to my work email address. 'You haven't been in touch for ages, I just want to make sure that everything's okay!' was his pained lament.

I showed it to a friend at work, who was always keen to hear about my latest man-related escapades. She advised me to continue ignoring him.

'Psycho,' she said.

I sighed. 'He seemed really nice though.'

My colleague laughed. 'A nice psycho is still a psycho.'

*

My UK visa came through in ten days. I booked my flights. I was going travelling through the United States and Canada for nearly three months and would arrive in London at the start of July. The timing was most fortuitous; Ironman, Louise and I had been given notice to vacate the Fairfield house at the start of April because the landlord had decided to sell. It was perfect – one less thing to worry about. Everything was coming together.

Goodbye, Melbourne; hello, world

I had underestimated how hard it was to pack up your entire life, and to do it on your own. Now that my time in Melbourne was coming to an end, everything felt different, like Hobart had been once Glenn and I had made the decision to leave. My bedroom was being dismantled piece by piece. The house was filled with boxes. All the debris from my marriage couldn't just stay in the garage any more so I spent an entire Sunday going through it with a Missy Higgins album on repeat. By the end of the day, the pavement outside the house was crowded with hard waste, remnants of a life that only reflected how innocent I'd been, and how little idea I'd had of my taste, my identity, other than what I had poured into Glenn.

I was not sorry to see any of it go. I sold my furniture and white-goods on eBay; the leather couch Glenn and I had picked out together when we were newly engaged went to a B&B in Marysville, the dining table to a guy in Sandringham, the chest freezer to Louise's parents in St Andrews. My possessions were now scattered, in new homes and hopefully being put to new purposes. Only things that I loved and valued would be travelling with me. Everything else would be going back to Mum and Dad's in Hobart, where they had offered to store boxes for me in their spacious garage. I had packed up two boxes containing things I thought I might need in England – a portable electric heater, a favourite teapot, clothes, bedding, a few treasured trinkets. And books. Everything else I was leaving.

Having felt restless and unhappy there for a few months, I hadn't expected leaving Melbourne to be so difficult. I felt like I was attending a party and a funeral all at once. It was difficult to know where I stood with people. When I first announced I was officially leaving, my social life dropped dead and I spent more time alone than I had in years. I felt a bit sad and forgotten about, as if I had already gone. But now, with only a few weeks until I was due to fly out, it was as if my friends suddenly remembered I existed and I was being dragged in twenty different directions.

'I'm either the most popular girl in the world, or I'm all alone,' I lamented to Jules at one of our last sessions, sipping the familiar brown rice tea. 'My conscience is either nonexistent, or it's a lead weight. Why does my life have to be lived in such extremes? It's exhausting!'

Jules smiled a knowing smile. 'Philippa, it actually isn't. The problem is that you're allowing what other people want and how they treat you to be paramount in your emotional wellbeing. Switch off from it. You don't have to be everything to everyone. You're leaving. This is your choice. You can't please everyone, so you might as well do what you want.'

I was sorry my work with Jules was coming to an end. She had been so kind, and had encouraged me so much to move forward. At the end of our last session, she wished me well with my travels and told me that she believed in me. 'It's been a real privilege to be a part of your journey,' Jules said warmly as we hugged for the last time. She held me away from her and smiled like a proud aunt. '*Namaste.*'

There were some other wonderful moments in the midst of all the weirdness of leaving. Autumn now had a grasp on Melbourne, filling the air with its chilly breath, and the streets were thick with fallen leaves. I ran most mornings, breathing in the scent of the bush by the Yarra trail. Drove in my soon-to-be-sold car, singing Kelly Clarkson's 'Since U Been Gone' and Gloria Gaynor's 'I Will Survive' at the top of my lungs. Had Ashley and her baby girl round for a farewell picnic on my back deck at Casa de Ironman. We ate all kinds of goodies from the Queen Vic Market – cheese, bread, olives – and then it had started to rain lightly. I leaped up, assuming Ashley would want to take the baby inside. But she had remained where she was, in her deckchair, holding her daughter on her lap.

'It's just a bit of rain, it's not going to hurt her,' Ashley said, smiling. 'I don't want her to be afraid of life. I want her to feel things.'

I was so sad to say goodbye to Ashley. While we didn't see as much of each other these days, my friendship with her hadn't changed like so many of the other blogging friendships had recently.

She had been a rock for me and had always been so kind. Once, when I first moved to the city and told Ashley how I was missing my sisters back in Hobart, she had put a comforting arm through mine and said, 'I'll be your Melbourne sister.' Indeed she was, and she still is.

Then there had been a farewell party in a beachfront bar. Pretty much every weight-loss blogger in Melbourne turned up for it, as well as other friends and workmates, and even Ironman, who I think was amused and bewildered that so many people at the party knew who he was. We ended up all over St Kilda that night, first in a backpacker's nightclub, then in a sex shop (which was a huge laugh) and then finally nibbling on late-night sugary treats from one of the cake emporiums on Acland Street.

I remember sitting there with my friends as we ate our indulgences, finding that I was satisfied with a few mouthfuls. I had stopped counting points many months earlier, when I had had many other things on my mind. I had still been dropping the kilos anyway, with very little effort on my part, so I figured I might as well ease off and see how I went. It turned out I was able to exercise portion control without the structure of a points or calorie counting system, and I was also able to eat intuitively, something I'd never been able to do before. I had reached a natural place where I allowed myself to have pretty much whatever I wanted, provided I had checked in with my emotions and found I had genuine hunger or a desire for a treat, rather than just dealing with uncomfortable feelings. I finally trusted myself not to go overboard and even if I did indulge, I was now so active that I could burn it all off anyway. For the first time in my life, food had been the least of my worries. Now it was just something I genuinely took pleasure in, with no guilt whatsoever.

*

Finally, the day dawned. Everything was sold and gone, or packed. Everything of value was in my rucksack. I had never felt more free or more terrified. By the time the plane pulled away from the gate and soared into the sky, I let it sink in that I was gone. I thought about all the goodbyes, all the pieces of my life as I knew it falling away. My time in Melbourne, which had been the setting of so many significant events in my life for the past year, was over.

My few days in Hobart with my family were lovely but turned sour with the sudden onset of tonsillitis. I doped myself up on medicine and tried to make the most of it. We celebrated my youngest nephew's first birthday (on Anzac Day, which meant that I had been at goal for a year!) but I couldn't eat any cake; my family took me to Fish 349 in North Hobart for a farewell dinner of sorts, and trying to eat was like swallowing razorblades. Anne took me out for afternoon tea at Hadley's and I sat there, a scarf around my neck, draining the pot of tea and picking at the scones. It still amazed me how much socialising revolved around food. We had a wonderful time, reminiscing about how much life had changed, and Anne's own tales of her travels got me excited and nervous in equal measure. At this stage I'd be lucky if I even survived the flight with my eardrums in tact. I shuddered and felt like everything was aching with even the smallest movement.

When I left two days later, sated by penicillin, my eyes bright with both excitement and frightened tears, I hugged my parents and

Anne, who had come to see me off, in the familiar departure lounge of Hobart Airport. Both Mum and Dad appeared devastated. Mum's body shook slightly with sobs as she hugged me against her, my shoulder damp with her tears.

I was the last person on the plane.

American dream

When you've never been on a long-haul flight before, nothing really prepares you for it. I arrived in San Francisco dazed and exhausted, but the thrill of being somewhere new ensured my drooping eyes stayed open for as long as possible. By the time I came to write in my journal I had been gone from Australia for two days, but it was already tomorrow there, something I really couldn't get my head around. My body was aching with fatigue, my head felt constantly cloudy and yet my heart felt like it would explode with joy.

I stayed in a hostel on the fringe of the Tenderloin area – not the nicest part of town, but it was incredibly cheap, had a pancake station for breakfast every day, and was chock-full of eligible young men. Just what this lonely travelling single girl needed.

I spent a lot of time exploring the city on foot, up the enormous hills and down to the wharf, where I partook of all the San Franciscan culinary delights – clam chowder served in a sourdough bread bowl; double-doubles at In-N-Out Burger; every kind of chocolate known to man at Ghirardelli's; and the weird and wonderful comestibles of Trader Joe's, where I found peanut butter cups, blueberry crumpets and almond butter to stash in my dorm locker for late-night snacks. I also went to the farmers' market, where I bought the sweetest and juiciest strawberries and oranges I'd ever tasted. I visited Alcatraz, rode across the Golden Gate Bridge with two British university students I met at the hostel (who insisted on riding a tandem bike together and gave me the nickname 'Oz'), and took a bus to Haight-Ashbury, which I found intimidating. There were a lot of people on the street asking for drugs (or asking if I wanted to buy any, like one girl did the minute I got off the bus) and a homeless man who had a rabbit puppet on his hand, which was holding a real gun. He pointed it at people as they walked by. I was so freaked out. I had seen some bizarre things on the streets of Melbourne, but never anything as menacing as this. I caught the bus back to the city pretty much immediately, relieved to be heading back to a safer part of town. I was blown away by how enormous and sophisticated the department stores in San Francisco were. Bloomingdales and Neiman Marcus made David Jones look like a discount warehouse. I wore thongs everywhere, even though I was walking seven hours a day. 'Hey, girl! Let me shine them toes!' laughed the shoe-shine man in Union Square. It all blew my mind.

It was a strange feeling, this being cast adrift in a foreign country, feeling lost yet knowing I was one step closer to finding what it was I truly wanted. There was also the knowing it had all been my choice. I focused on the excitement more than the fear, but I had to get used to being scared.

Alone and lonely were also two things I needed to get used to being. In Melbourne I hadn't really allowed myself to feel either of those things, even with all the therapy I'd had. The past nine months had been an absolute feast, compared with the previous seven years, of flirting and attraction. Occasionally that had turned into a one-night stand, a short-term relationship or a fling that never went anywhere. I thought I was living it up and playing the field, but actually I was just doing whatever it took to feel better. I ached for a warm body next to mine, to feel adored and wanted, to help ease the shame and fear that the end of my marriage had actually been all my fault because I was fundamentally unloveable.

San Francisco was not the setting for this epiphany, however, and in my one week in that city, there were quite a few flirtatious adventures. I could have blamed the jet-lag, the excitement of being in a new country, the daily arrival of new handsome hostel guests, or my naivety in thinking that every encounter was going to lead to some great love affair, but ultimately, for a young woman who had spent most of her life up until the age of twenty-five feeling invisible and unattractive, the admiration and clear approval I was getting was like catnip. I didn't notice that, like most vulnerable people with a mood enhancer, I was sliding into addiction and, like all addicts, I now relied on the attention to feel good and was always thinking about the next hit.

Foolishly, I blogged (it was still password-protected) about one of my San Francisco encounters, in a jokey Mills & Boon–esque way. I wrote it to give people a laugh, really, as the incident had been very funny and a bit naughty (while still being safe, of course). To my shock, some of the comments I got on that post were rude and patronising, including one from Gillian, who had regaled me with so many of her own single girl tales, often far more risqué than mine ever were.

The judgement of others still cut deep. I didn't yet have solid enough self-worth to openly live a life centred around my own needs, physical or otherwise. It's sad how much judgement gets flung your way when you're a woman living purely for the moment, who allows her desires and urges to take centre stage, and how dangerous it can be to openly discuss them. I wrote the occasional post, as a single woman, about consensual sex, Brazilian waxes and vibrators, because I found it very empowering to do so. As a fairly inexperienced and newly single woman, I wanted to know what other women thought about these things, and while I can appreciate it was oversharing in many respects, I was surprised to find that it meant, to some of my readers, that I had no morals. I suppose my naivety combined with my sudden Samantha Jones–esque bravado was a strange cocktail. Some people drank it with gusto, others sipped politely, others spat it out. And even though after San Francisco I was going to be staying with a blogger or a reader in every city I was visiting, the blogging world still felt very small to me. I felt like I was writing for my friends. I tend to only read the blogs of people I like and whose writing I enjoy, but it was slowly dawning on me that not all of my readers necessarily had that same attitude. I decided to never write about any romantic encounter, however entertaining, again. It was clear I needed to be more discreet.

Well, this is what you wanted. Freedom, I thought to myself as I journalled in cafes and sat in bookshops, reading. I certainly had freedom now but where it was going to take me, I had no idea.

*

My next stop was Albuquerque, New Mexico, where I was going to meet up with Nicole, a devoted reader of my adventures, who had often left supportive comments or emailed me to offer her thoughts on my latest disaster or quandary. She had always been a voice of wisdom and I had enjoyed getting to know her over email in the past year. I had no idea what she looked like and as I wandered through the airport, which – with its terracotta-tiled floors, timber beams and white and turquoise patterned walls – was unlike any other airport I'd ever been to. I gathered my backpack from baggage claim and tried to find Nicole. I saw a woman I thought might be her, but wasn't sure, so I started sniffing around for a pay phone so I could call her. I fished out a few quarters and then felt a tap on my shoulder. It was the woman I'd thought was Nicole! We hugged joyfully. She was so bubbly and friendly and we got on famously, as I knew we would.

We drove out into Albuquerque, a spectacular city that left me breathless. It was very flat, but with stunning natural rock formations and lush greenery, and with the Sandia Mountains forming a backdrop for some of the bluest skies and fluffiest white clouds I had ever seen. Even the smell in the air was magic – desert sand, spring flowers and spices.

We arrived at Nicole's home, dropped my bags, had a glass of wine and talked for hours, about my trip and our lives. Nicole is a gifted woman with amazing intuitive abilities. I was blown away by some of the things she said to me that afternoon. She told me that this trip I was on, through America and Canada, was going to reveal the real me.

'Everywhere you go, another layer will be peeled off,' she said, smiling. 'By the time you get to London, you will be your real self. You won't want to hide it any more. Everything will fall into place there.' We talked a bit about my marriage breakdown and she told me a few things that were apparently going to eventuate in Glenn's life that made me laugh but also made me feel a bit sad. I could finally see that ending that marriage, as excruciating as it was, had been the kindest thing to do for both of us. Glenn deserved to be loved by someone who didn't need him to change. I wondered aloud if I would ever marry again.

'Of course you will,' Nicole said. 'That's a given. But you'll meet this person when you are content with your life and who you are. This person will come along and you'll think, *This wasn't part of the plan.*' I could only smile. It still felt impossible.

My ten days in Albuquerque really weren't enough. Every day Nicole and I did something fun together, whether it was taking a cable car up the mountains, driving out to the Jemez Pueblo, or exploring bookstores in the Rio Grande valley, where I bought Nicole a copy of *Eat Pray Love*, one of my favourite books, and Nicole gave me her old copy of a book I had longed to own for years, Natalie Goldberg's *Writing Down the Bones*. We had a girl's day out in Santa Fe, the hometown of Nicole's good friend Tammy, who had us round to her place one evening for what she called 'a God show'. It turned out she meant the sunset. She lived in a house at the foothills of the

Sandia peaks, where the views were incredible and the sunsets even more so. We drank wine and watched this beautiful sunset, streaking the sky every shade of pink and gold and flaming red. A lot of the time we hung out at Satellite Coffee, a wonderful neighbourhood coffee house, where I journalled and people-watched, drinking as many cinnamon- and chilli-laced Mexican lattes as my bloodstream would allow.

A few days into my stay, Nicole and I went for a road trip to the Bandelier National Monument, where we did a bit of hiking to burn off our green chilli cheeseburgers. We walked by a flowing creek. Nicole went over to the edge, knelt down and ran her hand through the water. I came over and did the same. 'When you try to hold water in your hand, it falls away so quickly,' she said. 'It's the same with love. Love isn't possession. You have to let it flow through you, around you, rather than try to hold on to it. The harder you try, the faster it falls away.'

I thought about that a lot. I didn't think I had been possessive with any of the men I had dated in Melbourne, but maybe I had. Maybe I had tried to hold on to them, even the ones who were blatantly unavailable, just to make myself feel better. Maybe even Glenn, in the last few months we had been married. I had hung on, too afraid to tell him I wanted out, because sticking it out made me feel less guilty.

'Every man you have been with has taught you something, Phil,' Nicole said. 'And you'll get tested again, to see if you've truly learned those lessons. But you'll get there. The main thing is that you keep learning from everything.'

I was truly overwhelmed by Nicole's kindness, by how she had welcomed me into her home and her life and made me feel so comfortable. When I came to my last night in Albuquerque I felt equally sad to be leaving my dear friend and thrilled to be taking the next step of the journey, the journey I was truly meant to be on, which would take me closer and closer to where I needed to be.

We met Tammy for a farewell drink in a coffee house near the university in the centre of town, where they were setting up for an open mic night. I was convinced by Nicole and Tammy to get up there and tell some of my travel tales, and ended up revealing the story of a strange outing I had been on a few days earlier, with a man I'd met while Nicole had been at work.

This man was a native Bostonian, transplanted to the midwest, who worked as a private investigator and had got my attention by dropping his keys in front of me while I was writing and sculling lattes at Satellite Coffee. He gave me his business card, which featured a photo of him twenty years ago on the front cover of *Police: The Law Officers Magazine*. He was incredibly friendly and didn't seem to be crazy, apart from being fascinated by my accent, which he'd initially mistaken for Texan. We arranged to meet the following day so he could take me to see Madrid, a charming little town about an hour out of Albuquerque. All the Americans I'd met so far had been very friendly, hospitable and keen to show me around, so I didn't think he had any ulterior motives – he was old enough to be my father. When we met up and I got in the car, I noticed he seemed to be having trouble getting it to start.

'Oh, wait just a second,' said Mr Texas (as Nicole and I now dubbed him), reaching down to his right. He pulled up a device and blew into it. It took him about three enormous blows but finally the car started. It suddenly dawned on me – it was a breathalyser! In New Mexico, he told me, if you are convicted of a drink-driving offence, your vehicle must be fitted with one of these devices for a year and if it detects any alcohol at all, the car won't start. They are so sensitive they even pick up mouthwash.

Mr Texas saw my face, which must have been somewhere between amused and horrified. 'Oh, it wasn't my fault; my lawyer really screwed up!' he said, telling me the whole story as we headed out towards Madrid. It was a very pleasant day and we had some nice talks, but I was relieved when he looked at his watch, which hinted that maybe the outing was at an end.

'Oh, shoot!' he exclaimed. 'I have to pick up my kids from school. It's on the way back to your place. Okay if we get them first?'

It wasn't like I could refuse, really, but I didn't want his kids thinking I was his new girlfriend. We picked up his son first, who was a very sweet twelve-year-old, and we talked pleasantly about his band, his lizard collection and what he wanted to do when he left school. His younger sister eyed me with great suspicion and didn't say a word to me. 'Must be freaked out by your accent,' was Mr Texas's thinking. As if that weren't awkward enough, the children announced they had left things at their mother's house that they needed, so we ended up stopping by the residence of the former Mrs Texas. I sank low into my seat, desperately hoping I wouldn't be seen, but I'm sure Mr Texas was hoping for the opposite. I'm happy to say Mr Texas and I parted as friends ... who would never see each other again.

And so I told this story on my last night in New Mexico to the appreciative crowd at the coffee house in downtown Albuquerque, who howled with laughter at some of it, particularly the breath-alyser part.

'Welcome to America!' called someone from the audience. It was awesome.

When Nicole and I finally returned to her place that night, she did a tarot reading for me – a tradition for all her guests, she said. She also told me what she could sense about my future husband. I was incredibly dubious about this, despite trusting her and her intuitive abilities, as she hadn't steered me wrong so far. For where I was in that moment, a sex change held more appeal than remarrying. But Nicole was insistent it would happen.

'I sense he's slightly older than you, with dark hair,' she said.

'He's not Australian, is he?' I asked, already knowing the answer.

'No. He's English.'

'Okay, tell me more,' I said, smiling. I thought I might as well hear it all so I could at least be on the lookout for this dreamboat once I landed in London.

'He's an ambitious guy, very artistic,' she said. 'He'll be involved in the theatre in some way. Maybe he's a playwright? I see writing of some kind, at least. In fact, very early on he will show you a book filled with things he's written, maybe even drawn. Like I say, artistic.' She paused, as if she were listening to someone. 'His grandmother is deceased. She's telling me that you just need to trust her and be patient, and she will take care of it all. She will make sure the two of you meet when you're both ready for it.'

As strange as this sounds, I believed her. While I maintained a healthy scepticism, my heart was slowly starting to hope again.

I didn't go to bed until 3.30 a.m. and had to be up again at 5 to catch my flight to Denver, Colorado. We stopped at Satellite Coffee on the way to the airport for my last Mexican latte. It was dark outside and the inside of the coffee house looked like a planetarium. The coffee was as warm, sweet and spicy with cinnamon and chilli as it had been every time I'd enjoyed one. Saying goodbye to Nicole was incredibly difficult but I knew I had made a friend for life and that we would see each other again. In the meantime, I was feeling enlightened and empowered, with a sense of clarity and calm that I hadn't had when I arrived. I knew now I had to trust the Universe and, more importantly, I had to trust myself. Everything would unfold as it was meant to.

*

My two days in Denver passed far too quickly in the company of blogger Andrea and her husband, Sean, who showed me a wonderful time. We went to a Rockies baseball game, visited The Tattered Cover bookstore, bar-hopped among some of Denver's best watering holes, and then went on a day-long hike in the Rocky Mountains, which finished with a catfish dinner and beers at the Oskar Blues Brewery. Andrea and Sean were truly delightful people who, like Nicole, felt like kindred spirits. I was sorry to leave so soon but excited to land in Vancouver, and curious to see how different Canada would be to what I'd experienced in America so far.

I waltzed up to the immigration desk at Vancouver Airport with my passport and a huge smile but the immigration official didn't seem thrilled that Philippa Moore wished to enter Canada.

He looked scornfully at the form I had just filled in. 'Why are you going to be in Canada for twenty-eight days, Ms Moore?' he asked dryly.

I explained I was on holiday and was going to be visiting friends.

'Who are these friends of yours? How long have you known them?'

I told him they were fellow bloggers and we had been corresponding for over a year. The official's eyes narrowed. 'So you've never met these people before?'

'Well, no,' I admitted, now starting to panic that I would never get to meet them. 'But I *know* them. We've talked on the phone, exchanged lots of emails and photos. I know what they look like.' God, even I thought I sounded dodgy now.

The official still looked sceptical and started asking me questions about Sarah and Brianna – who were they, where did they live, what did they do for a living. Some of those things I knew but others I had to make up. Finally, after I'd convinced myself I was not going to be allowed into Canada at all, he stamped my passport.

'Have fun,' he said, his face betraying nothing.

I finally got out into the arrivals hall, where poor Sarah and her fiancé, Dave, would now have been waiting for ages. I scanned the crowds for her friendly face.

'Phil!' she called out. I gave her as big a hug as I could manage with my giant backpack. I liked her and Dave immediately – it was, again, as if we were old friends. They had kindly arranged for me to housesit for one of their friends for the two weeks I'd be there, in a basement suite of a grand old house on Point Grey Road, owned by a couple in their nineties, Mr and Mrs Carter. The views from my 'basement' suite were stunning, with Stanley Park and Kitsilano

Beach to the right, the tall skyscrapers of Vancouver with imposing snow-covered mountains in the background and a sparkling ocean in front of me. My first meal in Vancouver was at the vegetarian institution The Naam. It was also my introduction to Sarah and Dave's lifestyle as environmentalist vegetarians, or what might have been known back in Australia as 'greenies'. We had incredible talks and everything they said made so much sense. I had flirted with vegetarianism many times growing up, but it was always met with a lot of opposition, which made me uncomfortable. But at this point in time, I had challenged an awful lot of my old behaviours, thoughts, patterns and habits, all of which I did purely because they were acceptable and familiar. Slowly but surely, everything in my life was coming under the microscope, particularly as I grew more comfortable with myself and who I was, and found I wanted to live a life that was more aligned with my values and beliefs, rather than just doing things to keep other people happy.

The thing about Sarah and Dave, and their families, was that they simply got on with the business of living the most conscious and ethical lives they could, doing everything in their control to bring about the change they wanted to see and the kind of world they wanted to live in. While they were happy to talk about it if asked, they did it quietly, without fanfare. It was so inspiring to see them living their lives around their values and beliefs without being obsessive about it. We had many long discussions about the devastating effect the meat industry has on the environment. It struck me that it was all very well for me to have made changes to make my own life better, but what about the wider world? I was enjoying a healthy and active lifestyle, but what about my ethics and values?

How was I living those? What did I stand for? If I was aware of food production practices I didn't agree with that were harming the planet, why was I supporting them by giving them my money and consuming the product? I won't bombard you with the stats – that isn't the point of this book – but I found them confronting and frightening, and discussing this with Sarah and Dave cemented my feeling that I wanted to be doing my bit, in whatever way I could.

On my first night in Canada, we caught the ferry out to Mayne Island to visit Dave's family, who were staying in their farmhouse there. It was also where Sarah and Dave were going to be married the following month. I met Dave's parents, Bill and Kris, and various members of his extended family, who often came to spend weekends at the farm.

'So, how do you know Sarah?' Kris asked me as we settled in with a glass of excellent red wine.

I had asked Sarah and Dave earlier whether we needed to come up with a less dodgy-sounding story than 'the internet', remembering the less-than-impressed immigration official who had only just let me into the country. But Sarah was confident it would be fine to tell the truth.

Kris frowned slightly when she heard the tale and looked at me with curiosity. 'So you've only met for the first time today?' she asked. She was a psychiatrist, so her gaze was not without its loaded meaning.

'That's right,' I said with a grin on my face, trying to sound as earnest and trustworthy as I could. It wasn't like I was a hitchhiker Sarah and Dave had just picked up! But a discussion ensued about how long had we known each other, what on earth a 'blog' was, how

Sarah had found mine, and how it was far more acceptable and common for people of our generation to meet over the internet – whereas for someone of Kris's age, the internet was still thought of as a dangerous place filled with swindlers and perverts. I felt her eyeing me with a little suspicion and I suppose I would have done the same in her position, but eventually she seemed to be won over. (Bless you, Kris.) The whole conversation reminded me that it *was* a strange but incredible thing that I, this ordinary Australian girl, had started a blog that had somehow found its way to the computer screen of another young woman in Canada. I was truly blown away by how far my little blog had reached and the wonderful people it had put in my path.

The next day, I was given a tour of the farm. There was an expansive organic vegetable garden with row after row of vegetables contained within animal-proof fencing. There were hammocks strung between the ancient gnarled trees, and the gardens were bursting with blue cornflowers and blood-red peonies. We walked through damp grassy meadows and over to the hill where Sarah and Dave were going to be married in less than four weeks' time. Finally we walked down to the pond and through an orchard filled with apple, pear and hazelnut trees, back to the house. It was some kind of paradise.

After we got back, Dave had a nap and Sarah and I curled up on the comfy couches in front of a roaring fire with mugs of hot tea and talked for ages. Thanks to my blog she knew a lot about me but I wanted to learn all about her, and over the next few hours I did. I felt very close to her. It was hard to believe I had only met her in person not even twenty-four hours prior.

The three of us made dinner before we headed off to catch the late ferry back to Vancouver. I made a tomato, cucumber and yoghurt raita and then sat down to write in my journal while Sarah and Dave made rice and dhal. I stopped writing at one point and just watched them. They were just preparing a simple meal together and yet I saw so much more – how well they worked as a team and how much they appreciated each other. At that moment I had a crystal-clear realisation of why my marriage to Glenn had never worked – we had never been a team. Sarah and Dave, by contrast, were so happy in each other's company and so kind to each other. Theirs was a true partnership, of shared ideals and dreams. I watched them together and thought, *This is what I want.*

Vancouver felt like an adopted hometown almost immediately. I went for daily walks and runs to Stanley Park and along the Kitsilano waterfront, tried out free classes at yoga studios, shopped for groceries in the local markets. I also met up with another online friend who was the first blogger I had ever read. I first found her blog in 2004 while I still worked in finance, bored and longing for adventure and space and time to pursue the things I really wanted to do. Brianna was a young writer who, at that point in time, had just quit a corporate job to focus on her writing, which was exactly what I wanted to do. Her life seemed to be everything that mine wasn't – authentic, purposeful, fulfilling, creative. The utter joy that came through in her words from following her passion, the tiny details in her everyday life like the steam rising from her morning coffee or the walks she took along the beach, and not to mention her actual writing itself, was utterly enthralling. And she was my age. It was a breath of fresh air that I had sorely needed. Eventually, after about a year of reading her blog, I left a comment for her on a post and then sent an email, introducing myself, pretty much spilling out everything that had changed in my life since finding her website and what I was hoping for in the future. She wrote back. And we've been friends ever since, just as I thought we would be.

Brianna and her husband, Mike, met me for dinner at The Eatery, a fabulous sushi restaurant a couple of blocks away from 'my' apartment. I felt like I was going to meet a character out of my favourite book. For so long, I'd read about and pictured Bri working away on her novel, in her kitchen making croissants, or walking in a market on her travels in Central America, and now here she was, sitting opposite me in a restaurant. It was bizarre, but incredibly wonderful. We talked effortlessly about life, travel, writing, love and everything in between. She and Mike were a lot like Sarah and Dave – very in tune with each other's needs, desires and goals in life. It gave me a great deal of hope that perhaps such a relationship was in my future too.

Vancouver was certainly a city of kindred spirits. Brianna and I went swimming, shopping and out for drinks, and I also hung out with Sarah nearly every day and grew to absolutely adore her. She and Dave took me to a cabin in Whistler for a few nights, where we enjoyed hikes and fun evenings in with wine, Bear Claw ice-cream and board games. The day we drove back to Vancouver was my twenty-sixth birthday. We had plans to meet up with Brianna and Mike that night for drinks and birthday cupcakes but Sarah and Dave had a few wedding errands to run in the afternoon so I was left to my own devices for a few hours. I went to The Naam by myself for coffee and a slice of birthday cranberry and apple pie, and pulled out of my bag something I had found when packing up Casa de

Ironman a few months earlier. It was a letter I had written to myself in 1997 at age sixteen, to be opened on my twenty-sixth birthday. I was amazed curiosity had never got the better of me over the years.

I broke the seal that had been there for ten years and read the familiar handwriting, far neater than mine was now. I smiled and laughed out loud at some of it, but there were things I'd written – naive, innocent things – that made me want to put my head on the scarred wooden table in that crowded cafe and weep. 'Are you married yet?' 1997 Phil had asked. 'I always have fantasies of getting married.' Oh dear. The whole tone of the letter made me sad, remembering the girl who wrote it; the girl who muddled her way through a world that confused and scared her; who made decisions based on zero confidence and an inability to see her worth, blindly following a fantasy. I pulled out my journal and pen and wrote a letter back to her, answering all her questions. It took some time. I was so glad to have moved on from that time, but I knew I was still dealing with the fallout.

Before I knew it, it was my last day in Vancouver. This was definitely the hardest goodbye so far. I hugged Sarah and Dave and thanked them for a wonderful time, trying hard not to cry.

'This isn't goodbye,' Sar said, squeezing my hand. 'We'll see each other again.'

You'd think with all the goodbyes I'd said recently I would have been used to them, but parting was always a bit difficult. Fortunately the pain was always fleeting; it always dissipated once I moved on to the next adventure. I missed people, of course, but there was something greater pushing me along on that journey, something that kept making me put one foot in front of the other.

My next stops were Toronto and Montreal. I stayed with a blog reader, Krissie, in her apartment on the fringe of Little Poland in Toronto, where you could hear the streetcars *ding-dinging* along the roads, and in Montreal I spent a rather glorious week with another blogger, Teresa, and her family, who were all keen that I enjoyed everything that lovely city had to offer.

Reading through my travel journals, interestingly it's in Montreal that the tone markedly changes, as if I found my real voice somewhere on those quaint cobbled streets in the Latin Quarter or at the bottom of an iced latte in Second Cup.

'This trip has changed me,' I wrote. 'I no longer feel the need to lay myself out there in the world, right down to the bones, raw, exposed. I need to protect myself. I've worked too hard to find myself to start giving myself away again.'

This need to protect myself had already meant, ironically, no more password-protected blogging; I had stopped that as I'd felt less comfortable putting so much of myself out there. I had a nagging feeling that I had been a bit naive and too trusting of people. Now my blog was public again. I kept it going because it was a good way to keep family and friends updated with what I was up to, and I still enjoyed writing it and getting nice comments (as well as travel tips) from my readers. But I didn't feel as safe talking about my private thoughts. Many times I went onto my blog and put on a brave face when I was desperate to tell the ugly and messy truth.

I enjoyed spending time with Teresa and her family, who made me feel so at home in Montreal. As had been the case everywhere I had been on the trip, my departure date rolled around far too quickly.

Teresa's husband drove me to the train station and gave me a warm hug as we said goodbye.

'You are very, very brave,' he said solemnly.

A few people had said that to me on the trip. In fact 'brave' was the adjective people used most frequently to describe me when commenting on my blog as well. It wasn't something I was consciously choosing to be, weirdly; I was just allowing what I wanted to be stronger than the fear of it all backfiring on me somehow. Admittedly, some days on the trip had been harder than others and I had felt very lonely at times. The reality of what had happened only a year earlier often hit me, especially when I hung out with lovely couples whose relationships were based on trust, mutual respect, shared passions and equality. It made me realise what a sham my marriage to Glenn had been. It had been a place for me to hide my fears and inadequacies. I actually began to feel quite sorry for him. How was he to know I had needs and desires when I had never expressed them? My focus had always been on keeping him happy, in exchange for his love, which in turn would feed my non-existent self-esteem. In my sad and lonely moments I wondered, was this all my fault? Could I have been happy with him and I had just thrown that possibility away because of my selfish needs?

I knew deep down that wasn't true. It wasn't like I hadn't tried to be happy with him, but I now knew in my heart that what I had experienced in my marriage was certainly not happiness. I had learned the true meaning of happiness on this trip, once I was free, once I was myself, for the first time. My heart had overflowed with love everywhere I went, for my new American and Canadian friends, and my friends back home, who had been kind, encouraging and generous; for my family, who I missed dearly; and for myself, for being, as many people pointed out, so brave. Somehow I had dug deep and made the life I so desperately wanted happen. I was starting to understand that this was how people healed. You eventually have to stop wallowing, stop going over the details of your heartbreak, and start running towards the life you *do* want. This is what I tell people now. No matter how bad things get, you must start moving towards the future. You can't look behind you; you can only look forwards. You have to keep going.

And now it was time for the next stop: New York City. I had planned to go to a hostel but Lola, a friend in Queens, had unexpectedly and very kindly offered to host me, and so it was arranged that I would meet her in a bar once she finished work that evening. I boarded the train that left Montreal at 9 a.m. It took nearly thirteen hours to reach Penn Station, longer than it had taken to fly from Sydney to San Francisco, not helped by a two-hour delay at the Canadian/US border. It was such a relief to finally get there after sitting in the cramped chair all day. I had expected to feel frightened and overwhelmed, but instead I was so excited as I emerged onto 34th Street. I saw Macy's, the bright glittering lights, the streets crammed with honking cars and hotdog carts. The air smelled like pretzels, spun sugar and fire. I stepped into the road, feeling like Carrie Bradshaw, and hailed my first yellow cab.

New York City was both everything and nothing like I thought it would be. It was completely unlike anywhere else I'd been in America. Everything was so surreal; I felt like I was on a movie set. Chance encounters in coffee shops or bars would lead to a night of dancing with strangers, or a motorbike ride across the city at midnight, my arms wrapped around a gorgeous off-duty NYPD officer. I got attention and validation everywhere I went in that city, but it wasn't enough any more. My heart was aching and I was tired of dating. Despite everything Nicole had told me in Albuquerque, I was beginning to think my search for love was permanently road-blocked. It would probably be years before I met the man she had told me about, which was fine, I was certainly in no hurry to settle down again, but what was I meant to do in the meantime?

Danger came in many disguises in New York City. I had been offered a modelling job – yes, I can actually hear you sighing right now! Of course the photographer would turn out to be a lecherous fuckwit with nothing but dishonourable intentions! But I had spent my childhood dreaming of being 'discovered', so I felt compelled to give it a shot, and my friend Lola, a model herself, thought the offer seemed genuine too. My childhood dream very quickly became something else; that photo shoot in a New Jersey warehouse was one of the most skin-crawlingly unpleasant experiences I've ever had. He was a legit photographer – the studio was crammed full of ad campaigns he'd shot previously – but as I started posing it became very clear that this photographer had other things in mind. Every advance I rejected was followed by another. He was a man who was very used to getting what he wanted. It dawned on me, as he pressed me to the ground and tried to stick his tongue into my mouth, that I was unsafe and needed to manage the situation, so I deployed my gift of the gab. I asked him questions about himself so his other brain would kick into gear. I remembered some things he had said about his mother and sister earlier that night, so I asked about them. Reminding him of women in his life who he cared about and presumably would never want treated like this seemed to help him back off a little. I was lucky (though it's sad I have to use that word) that nothing else happened because it so easily could have. I felt very stupid. I got back to Lola's apartment in the early hours of the morning, having finally escaped, and stayed in the shower for ages, scrubbing every inch of my skin. Even though nothing else had happened I still felt violated. At a grotty Greek restaurant in Queens the next night, I told Lola and her friend Nick, a spin instructor who I'd also got to know in my time in the city, the entire humiliating tale in between bites of lemon potatoes and vegetarian moussaka. The photographer had been trying to call me all day – at least thirty missed calls were racked up in my phone log and I'd ignored every one. I was feeling very down about the whole thing.

'You looked so pretty too,' said Lola, who had helped me straighten my hair for the shoot. 'I wonder if you'll ever see any of the pictures?'

'That's if there was any film in the camera,' Nick said, laughing. 'I'll bet there wasn't!'

I was so embarrassed. Of course the photographer had had an ulterior motive – no one in their right mind would offer me a modelling job. I was hardly Elle Macpherson. Why hadn't I twigged? Nick and Lola were very kind and assured me I had no reason to feel embarrassed – I'd walked away unharmed, with a tale to tell, and in a big city like New York such incidents were not uncommon, sadly.

'In this city,' Nick explained, 'it's either about ass, or money, or possessions. People try to separate you from your shit as fast as possible. It's Scam City, USA.' He laughed. 'Think you'll come back?'

'I hope so,' I replied. I meant it, despite everything.

My next, and penultimate, stop was Annapolis, Maryland. Lola and Nick tried to convince me to stay in New York, telling me they would help me find an apartment and a job. I'd already been offered a job, actually – by the photographer, to be his assistant. But even I wasn't that stupid. I was going to see my friends Valerie and Jim, who I had met on their own trip to Australia some six years before. I had stayed in touch faithfully with Val, a writer of some renown, and I fell into her arms at the train station like those six years had been merely weeks.

When we got to their house, Jim had all the fixings for one of his famous gin and tonics out on the porch. By now, summer had well and truly arrived so we sat on their porch in the early evening heat, sipping ice-cold drinks while excellent jazz purred from their stereo. Jim was a musician, as well as a writer, psychologist and member of the first American expedition to Mount Everest in the early 1960s, so he and Val regaled me with wonderful stories through-out my visit. It was like I was staying with family. It felt comfortable and familiar and was a much-needed respite from the relentless highs and lows of New York. I slept under an Amish quilt, went hiking and kayaking with Jim, attended barbecues and firework parties with the neighbourhood twenty- and thirty-somethings. Val showed me some of her novel in progress and I showed her some short stories I had been working on. Her critiques were kind but firm – I needed to push the boundaries in my work as much as I was in reality. 'Do with your writing what you're doing with your life,' Val advised sagely. 'Be brave.'

Finally I reached the last stop, Washington DC, from where I would fly to London. It was very cosmopolitan and also surprisingly easy to find my way around. I spent hours wandering around the art galleries and the National Library of Congress, and sitting in the blazing heat by bubbling fountains, cooling my feet and relieving the oozing burn I had on my ankle from the motorcycle ride in New York City. Val and Jim's friend Julia was hosting me, and we did fun, girly things in the evenings once she finished work. On 4 July, we did a bike ride from her home on the outskirts of Georgetown to Mount Vernon, the home of George Washington, a 60 kilometre round trip. I hadn't got on a bike since my last triathlon, and I was surprised by and thrilled with my stamina. I enjoyed Julia's company; she too loved to travel and have adventures, and she really understood what I had faced and was facing and the desire to live a full and authentic life. The day ended in the Mall watching the jaw-dropping fireworks. It felt like a fitting end to my North American odyssey, the journey that had revealed so much, brought me lifetime friends, stripped away everything I thought I was and given me so much more. But Nicole's words were firm in my memory: 'London is where it will all come together.'

All change, please, all change

As my plane flew over London and I saw my new home from the air for the first time, I felt every single part of me tingle with joy. This was a part of the world I had longed to see for as long as I could remember, and finally I was there. It felt like a homecoming, as strange as that sounds. I wandered off the plane into Heathrow in a happy daze, following my fellow passengers down corridors that led to the passport queue. After my experience in Vancouver, I was armed with the answer to every possible question a hostile immigration officer might have. In the end the immigration officer took a cursory glance through my passport and then quickly stamped it.

'Welcome to the UK,' she said, smiling.

Considering this was where I was going to settle and live for the foreseeable future, I had never had less of a plan in my life. My plan was like a pay-as-you-go SIM card – I thought I would whack a bit of credit on and see how I went, perhaps reevaluate when the credit ran out.

As it happened, it ran out very quickly. London and I didn't get off to the best start. This was the last thing I expected. There was such a magic about the place – I loved the jugs of Pimm's in sweet character pubs; the green spacious parks that people flocked to on a summer day like you would a beach back home in Australia; the amazing markets full of vintage treasures; the libraries, theatres and bookshops I'd only ever dreamed about; the wonderful yoga studio that I started visiting daily; the rows of houses in Notting Hill that looked like sugared almonds. I walked the streets as if I had been walking them my whole life. There was something so natural about living in London for me. But when it came to the business of settling into this new country, things were trickier than I expected.

My childhood friend Vivienne, transplanted from Sydney to London some years before, was very generous and let me stay with her in her room in a large flat in a Bayswater mansion block that she shared with five other expats. The flat itself had five bedrooms and there were usually up to eight people there at any one time, a mixture of permanent residents and visitors. Vivienne, who had picked up a weird plummy accent since I last saw her, couldn't do enough for me and made me very welcome; some of her flatmates, however, made it clear that my stay couldn't be extensive. This was in harsh contrast to the hospitality I'd received on my travels so far. Today, having lived in London for some time, I understand the density of the place. Flats are small and there simply isn't the room to house travellers and new arrivals indefinitely as there is in spacious American and Australian homes. You get on top of each other very quickly. I can now well understand why yet another antipodean arrival would have put the other flatmates on edge. So there was no time to sit around – I had to find my own place as soon as possible.

I was employed within two weeks, as a production assistant at a publishing company, which was very exciting, but I wouldn't get a pay cheque straight away (salaries are paid monthly in the UK) and the search for a permanent home proved incredibly difficult. I had no idea where to start looking so I simply tried everything. I scoured *TNT Magazine*, trawled Gumtree, begged every contact I had. Before I knew it, it was the start of August and I had been in the UK for a month.

Angela was still planning to visit in September and stay with me. *Where?!* It would be sleeping bags under Waterloo Bridge at this rate. Eventually I came clean to her and explained the situation, which I had suspected might happen all along. I told her it was fine with me if she still wanted to come but as I had nowhere for her to stay she would have to make her own accommodation arrangements. She did not take this very well.

I had more pressing worries, however. Having become familiar with rejection over the past year, I was experiencing it on a whole other level with my London flat hunt. I kept a spreadsheet of the flats I viewed and the number was creeping up to forty. Every time I went to a viewing, I felt like an actor going for an audition. How well did I play the part of potential housemate? Was I keeping all my quirks and flaws suitably under wraps? I had to pick up on subtle cues from my fellow players – did they want a 'life of the party' girl or someone who kept to herself? Occasionally I would find a part I was convinced I could play. My potential housemates were lovely and welcoming so I would stay well past my allotted time, have a drink with them, and leave with the assurance I was the frontrunner but they still had a few people to see and it wouldn't be fair to cancel on them, much as they liked me. They would call. They promised.

If, after a few days, I hadn't heard anything, I would mark that place as red in my spreadsheet and move on. Only one place was courteous enough to ring and tell me I hadn't got the room. The girl who rang said they met about five people they really liked, including me, and in the end they simply put the names in a hat. It was little consolation. Was my name ever going to be drawn?

At first I had been quite picky about the places I considered. They were tiny, for a start, and very expensive. I had shared a three-bedroom, two-bathroom house in Melbourne for a measly $550 a month. On inspecting a cupboard-sized room in Brick Lane whose single window had an enticing view of a graffitied wall, I was told it was £700 a month – around $2000 at the time. I had to give up on the more exciting areas of London and research Zone 2 and 3 options. But the further out of the centre I went, the weirder people got. There was the landlady in Leytonstone who gave me the wrong directions and didn't answer my phone calls as she was still passed out from the night before. The landlord who could have walked right out of a Mike Leigh play and who, when I asked why there was no shower in his Swiss Cottage boarding house, said, 'Oh, there's a gym down the road. You can have a shower there.' In my desperation, I almost took that one.

And then there was the viewing in West Kensington, arranged via email with someone named Lauren. I found the address and knocked on the door. It was answered by a rugged Kiwi chap. When I announced who I was and that Lauren was expecting me, he gave me a vacant look and said, 'There's no Lauren living here.' I showed him the email print-out with the address on it, which confirmed I was in the right place, but the woman I had arranged to meet didn't exist. I don't know whether the room had already been let and rather than tell me that, they had made something up, or whether the real Lauren had just mistyped the address. Eventually I caught the bus back to Bayswater, trying not to cry. What was I going to do?

I had well and truly outstayed my welcome in Vivienne's flat so tried to be there as little as possible, which meant leaving early every morning, eating breakfast at work, staying out late and on weekends either sitting in the park if the weather was fine or in the library when it (usually) wasn't. I was barely eating. I subsisted on porridge and communal fruit and biscuits in the office and rarely bought a proper lunch because I was trying to spend as little as possible. I was paying for my spot at Vivienne's place by buying her dinner and drinks any time we went out, as well as making contributions when I could to her flat's 'kitty' for bills and the like, so my limited funds were dwindling. I needed to make sure I kept enough to cover the first month's rent and bond when I eventually did find a place, so a bed at one of London's obscenely priced hostels wasn't really an option. As a result, I had to trespass on my friend's kindness far longer than I would have liked. Every evening I'd have three or four flat viewings lined up all over the city. I was exhausted all the time and I'd dropped a few more kilograms, but this time that wasn't a good thing. I knew I couldn't continue like this but every day my search for a home in this mad, hectic city seemed to grow more and more fruitless.

At this point, I considered the strong possibility I would have to go home to Australia. But what would I go back to? When I thought of everything I had given up to be in London – my job, my friends, my family, not to mention all the money I'd spent – it made me want to be sick. I was tired of being a nomad and was longing to settle in properly and for my new life in London to get started. I didn't feel I could tell anyone the truth about how tough I was finding things either. My family, approachable as they were, would only worry. As it was, Dad had read my latest blog post, in which I'd been my typical over-dramatic self and had phoned me immediately, attempting to talk me off the metaphorical ledge. I told my friends in London as much as I dared – they were all sympathetic but unable to help, and I didn't want to complain to Vivienne too much, as she had been generous enough. Many of my blogging friends back in Melbourne had gone strangely quiet. I still heard regularly from Meredith, but it was mostly to tell me how upset Angela was with me about her cancelled visit.

I felt utterly adrift. I had thought London was where 'it will all come together' and therefore everything should have fallen into place by now. Looking back, that was a rather foolish and entitled thing to think. I had conveniently forgotten that not everything had been an uphill struggle – I had found a good job very easily and had certainly found my feet socially, making lots of new friends. As usual, I was focusing on the one thing that hadn't gone right, but having no permanent home yet was a lead weight and something I found very stressful. I sought help from every direction but the Universe was clearly telling me this was something I had to sort out by myself.

Which was, of course, exactly what I needed.

*

I left the Bayswater flat and went to doss with another friend in the Elephant and Castle area. They had someone else arriving to stay in ten days so I couldn't stay there indefinitely either; I had to stop being fussy and just get a room, a roof, anywhere. Anything that was cheap, rat-free and in Zone 2, I saw. But there was still nothing. London was testing me, not just in my search for a home, but in the continuing natural disaster that was my love life. Every man I went on a date with turned out to have major issues, and not of the girl-friend variety à la Cab Rank: they were just strange. I didn't even know how I ended up eating risotto across from them, the passable white wine numbing the awkwardness. And whenever I decided I actually liked someone, *poof*, they'd disappear, just like any pros-pects of London working out for me any time soon.

It wasn't just in gastro pubs or noisy bars that things got awk-ward with men in London. One evening, travelling to a flat viewing on the Northern line, I was listening to my iPod and trying to zone out. A funky song came on and, without thinking, I did a bit of a dance on the spot, a little hip shake. It was hardly a lap dance, but it prompted the man next to me to move closer and start bumping and grinding up against me. I was so shocked I got out at the next stop, breathless and teary and trying to calm myself down. I felt so dirty and cheap, like I had done something wrong. All I'd been

219

doing was enjoying my music and that had given this stranger free reign to objectify me.

Sometimes I thought that life was simpler when I'd been overweight. No one had paid me any attention. I'd been invisible, not a threat to anyone. My friends hadn't resented me for attracting attention when I went out with them, because I had never got any. I had been safe. Now I was visible and it was frightening.

I still loved London, despite everything. Something was pressing me to stay, even though things hadn't exactly been smooth sailing so far. But I started to understand why it was testing me so much. It was a crowded place, swamped with starry-eyed people like me who flocked to its shores every day. Every expat I'd met had some kind of settling-into-London horror story and I was starting to realise that London challenged people. It had to. If it was too easy, the city would be so crowded it would be uninhabitable. It had to make it hard so that those who had come there on a whim would be disheartened and give up, and only those with the strength and tenacity you need to survive there would keep going.

I started to think of London as a bit like me. I'd got a lot of attention in the past year or so, more than I'd ever got in my life, and while I believed most of it was genuine, I was beginning to understand that a lot of it had come from people who simply wanted a slice of the action, to soak in my new confidence, zest for life and belief, despite everything, that life was pretty fantastic. They wanted to shine in my light rather than seek their own. I had been learning, often the hard way, that sometimes you had to put up boundaries and that meant disappointing people. I hated that idea, admittedly, but I was beginning to see how allowing access to all areas of myself all the time (and not just in the obvious way) meant my body and soul were becoming uninhabitable, as indeed a city overrun with too many dreamers does.

I wrote a poem about this idea, called 'To London', and, after a bit of polishing, decided to take a punt and send it to *Smoke*, a literary magazine I'd spied on the counter at Foyles in Charing Cross Road. A week later, I had an email from the editor accepting it for publication in the next issue. If anyone wanted to see a young woman on top of the world, all they had to do was look at me. It was the moment things began to turn around.

The endless auditions for the role of ideal housemate continued until, at long last, I was told the front bedroom of a dilapidated five-bedroom house in Clapham North was mine. I would be sharing with two Australian girls and two blokes – one Australian, one Kiwi. I loved the room I was going to take over, which had a gorgeous mantelpiece over the (non-working) fireplace and a desk in the corner. There was an Australian flag pinned up in the hallway and a faded twig with gum leaves and gumnuts sticky-taped to the window above the front door, signifying it was Expat Central. It was an old house that was slowly falling apart – heavy rains once autumn hit would reveal a leak in the roof – but I was beyond being picky by then. The Friday I moved in I went back to the Bayswater flat after work to collect my boxes, which I could finally unpack after taping them up in Melbourne many months prior.

There was no lift so I got all my boxes down the six flights of stairs on my own. I had been warned that minicab drivers would charge extra if they helped with boxes so I stoically refused my cabbie's eager offer to help; the twenty-pound note in my wallet to pay for the ride was all I had on me. The driver was a little taken aback by my show of independence.

'You're a tough girl, aren't you?' he said. 'You come across like you really know how to look after yourself.'

'Well, I'm starting to,' I answered.

'Are you married, miss?'

I didn't know where that question had come from. Not 'Do you have a boyfriend?' but 'Are you married?'. Maybe, with all my bags and boxes, I looked like I was fleeing a marital home. I looked down at my left hand. The white tan line had completely faded.

'Technically, yes,' I answered. We hadn't yet applied for the divorce. 'But in reality, no.'

The car purred onwards to Clapham and the cabbie's twenty questions continued. He thought it was terribly sad that my young marriage was over.

'Don't you think it's sad, miss?' he asked.

'Of course I do,' I replied. 'But if I thought about how sad it was all the time, I wouldn't be able to get on with my life.'

He gave me his thoughts on relationships, youth and life. 'Embrace boredom,' was one of his pieces of advice. 'We all need something steady and solid in our lives. Someone to come home to, eat Chinese on the couch with, go all night without saying a word to each other but being comfortable. That's what real life is.'

I had to admit that I did miss that sometimes. But life was so much more fun this way, being on the edge rather than safely in the middle.

'I'd have made you a good husband, miss,' the cabbie said, smiling. 'If it weren't for the fact I've been happily married for eighteen years!'

Finally, he left me at the house, after insisting on helping me inside with the boxes. I let him this time.

*

It felt incredible to have a home in London at last – to finally unpack; to make a bed with my own familiar bed linen; to wash my clothes, buy new towels and revel in their cleanliness; to cook a meal; to shut a door and be completely alone in a space that was just mine; waking up each day in my own bed. Such small, small things that I knew I would never again take for granted.

With my spare time no longer entirely monopolised with the flat hunt, my evenings and weekends were now mine. On Saturdays I would go to the British Library, where I now had a reader's card, to write all day. On Sundays, I would walk a few blocks from my new home to Brixton, where I had discovered a favourite cafe, and would sit with a book and a latte (not to Melbourne standards but drinkable). In the other direction there was the green and expansive Clapham Common, where I went running most evenings after work. This was my dream life. I felt so proud of myself for making it happen and for the first time I felt okay about everything that had unfolded in Melbourne, including the separation.

Much as I still longed to find a special person to share my life with, I had finally realised that finding such a person would be meaningless unless I learned to truly love my own company first. The feeling of always being on the lookout for my next conquest suddenly vanished from my life. It wasn't a priority any more. Instead, I was my priority. I spent my evenings with friends, with books and the beginnings of my novel, or just by myself, going for a run, cooking a delicious healthy meal and having an early night. I felt nourished on every level and realised I was doing all of it for myself; I wasn't relying on anyone else. I felt complete, nurtured and excited about life. I woke up every day with a spring in my step. This unfriendly, unyielding city that had rejected me so many times over the past two months was suddenly paradise. *Who needs a guy?* I thought. *I want to be single.*

Of course, it wasn't always that simple. The bleaker and less happy facts of the past year would on the odd occasion hit me like a tidal wave. I got very lonely at times. But I was starting to see these longings and urges for what they were – cravings that could easily be met with a healthier choice. The parallels with my weight-loss journey weren't lost on me. Instead of fighting my loneliness, I was learning to embrace it. Much as I missed the security and comfort of a long-term relationship, I knew that living my passions and following my dreams were the keys to happiness for me. If I was doing that, I would be fine. Everything else was a bonus.

I wrote constantly. I still blogged but not as often, as I turned my attention to other genres and enjoyed letting my imagination loose. When I did update the blog it was mostly about places I had visited. It had become a very different space to the one I had started nearly two years ago, full of low-point recipes and exercise logs. Most of my writing was now done off-line. I threw myself into writing a novel I'd had in my head for a few years, and with the publication of more poems in London journals my joy and confidence grew. My focus on what I wanted to achieve with my life grew more razor-sharp, and I knew I couldn't afford any distractions.

London and I had made up. Life was good. It was time to show the world what I was made of.

It's only the beginning

The first day of September, a Saturday, was spellbindingly golden and light. I had spent the day writing in the British Library, as had become my usual Saturday habit, and then made my familiar way to Vivienne's flat in Bayswater to get ready to go out for her birthday drinks, her third birthday-related celebration so far. I had hit a bit of a stride with my writing and would have been quite content to stay at home that night. However, another friend, who had organised the location for the drinks that evening, had unexpectedly had to go to Scotland so was relying on me to be the birthday girl's 'maid of honour', as it were, and despite being on my dating sabbatical, I didn't want to become a hermit. I still enjoyed being social, seeing and being seen. I knew that if I ever found myself in a relationship again, it would be for reasons other than avoiding loneliness.

Throughout my trip in North America, after hearing Nicole's wise counsel, I had forced myself to put up boundaries and not give myself away as easily as I used to. Being a born people-pleaser, if I knew someone wanted something from me it was usually guaranteed they would get it. I had to put these new beliefs and my new self-respect into practice. I decided I wanted someone who liked me for myself. Someone I didn't have to hide my intelligence and quirky, nerdy interests from. A companion to weather all life's storms with. Someone who understood me. Someone who was as passionate about writing, literature, theatre, music and art as I was. Someone with ambition, who felt things deeply, who was fiery and alive. Someone who wanted me to reach my full potential, and who I could help reach theirs. Someone who was kind and gentle, who cared about the world. Someone who loved life.

But such a person wasn't on the horizon as far as I could see, and in the meantime I wasn't going to settle for anything less. While I had said that to myself countless times while surveying the single scene in Melbourne over the last year, like a stable owner looking for their next Cup winner, this time I actually meant it.

Vivienne and I curled our hair, did our make-up and sauntered down to Beach Blanket Babylon, a rather popular celeb hangout in Notting Hill. The drinks were beautiful, with real frangipanis floating on their icy jewelled surfaces, but each one cost what I was earning per hour in my job. I sipped very slowly indeed. More people showed up and eventually the cocktails became too expensive for everyone, not just me, so we moved to another bar a few streets away on Westbourne Grove. I sat with a cheap bottle of beer, sipping it at a snail's pace as I'd already spent too much money that night. I was feeling a little tired so I thought I'd finish my drink and then make my excuses.

If this were a movie, it would cut to a scene taking place on the other side of London, in a area south of the river called Battersea, where a young man named Tom had driven to the city that evening to crash with his older sister, a workmate of Vivienne's. Tom had recently returned from a year of travelling – to, fittingly, Australia – and was absolutely skint, so had just got a second job to keep himself going and pay off the credit card he'd used to pay for everything while he was Down Under, road-tripping through the Red Centre, getting his heart broken by his on again–off again Australian girlfriend, but generally having the adventure of his life. His second job was starting in a London auction house the very next day, so he was hoping to get an early night. But his sister, in her usual fashion, was flapping around getting ready for a birthday party she had been invited to. 'Why don't you come too? You might meet someone nice,' she said to Tom, angling for a lift – not only was she running late, she really didn't fancy bus-hopping through central London on a Saturday night, as no sane person would.

Tom was not enthusiastic. He had recently decided to take a break from dating. He'd spent the best part of a decade being jerked around and left hanging so he had decided to focus on getting his life back on track, finish writing a play he had been working on for a few years, maybe even go travelling again once he was earning decent money. No dating. He'd had enough.

But his sister wasn't going to take no for an answer and Tom was eventually cajoled into putting on a clean shirt and driving her across town to Notting Hill.

In the meantime, I had decided it was time to make my exit from the party before London's tubes turned into pumpkins. I gave Vivienne a hug and said I was going to head off. She pointed out her friend Zoë, who had just arrived and was standing at the bar. I had met Zoë once before, on my first weekend in London, when she joined Vivienne and me for a swim at the Serpentine, a lake in the middle of Hyde Park filled with ducks and slime, a popular spot in summer. We'd had a fun Sunday afternoon, lounging on deckchairs, eating strawberries and reading *Grazia*. I hadn't seen Zoë since, so I bounded over to say a quick hello. Those words had only just left my mouth when a rather handsome man with dark spiky hair sauntered up next to her. He looked at me with a curious smile.

'This is my brother,' Zoë said.

I stuck out my hand and smiled. 'Hi, I'm Phil.'

'I'm Tom,' he said, shaking my hand.

It turned out that originally Zoë had been left at the door by Tom, who had decided not to stay because it was now after 10 p.m. and the bar were enforcing a cover charge of ten pounds a head, which Tom didn't exactly have to spare – certainly not to gain admittance to a party he hadn't wanted to go to in the first place. He began to walk back to his car and had gone about a block when he heard someone running behind him. Convinced he was about to be mugged, he turned around. It was the bouncer.

'Mate, was it the birthday party you were going to?' he asked.

'Yeah, but I haven't got ten pounds to get in, sorry,' replied Tom.

The bouncer gestured back to the bar. 'No, don't worry, I'll let you in for free.'

That wasn't what he had expected to hear, in a city that's famous for being expensive. Tom, puzzled but pleased, went back to the bar and headed downstairs to the party.

I don't remember where our conversation went after that, but eventually Zoë's attention was elsewhere and we were the only two standing at the bar, chatting away, oblivious. I knew my plan to leave early had now gone out the window. I bought him a Coke, as we couldn't stand at the bar any longer without ordering something. Tom said later he felt he should have been more of a gentleman and bought me a drink, but based on his past experience with Australian women, he wasn't confident he'd ever see me again. As for me, I couldn't remember the last time I had enjoyed talking to someone so much. He was fascinating and we talked about all manner of things: travelling, theatre, Oscar Wilde, *The Simpsons*, writing, literature – all common interests and passions as it turned out. He was also employed, one of my main criteria after previous experiences. He had worked in IT for many years but was now a press officer for a regional theatre just outside of London.

'The pay is dreadful, as it tends to be in the arts,' he lamented, 'which is why I'm starting a second job tomorrow. I just didn't want to work in IT any more. It's not where my heart is. I love the theatre. I just decided I had to find a way to make it happen.'

When I think about meeting Tom, and our first conversation in that bar, the overwhelming feeling I remember is that it was like meeting an old friend, like I had known him for a very long time. Was it love at first sight? I didn't know it at the time, but looking back I think it was. What I did know was that while there was definitely a spark of some kind between us, I didn't feel nervous or desperate to impress him and say all the right things, as I had with other men I'd met in the past year. He put me immediately at ease. He had a wonderful smile, his eyes were twinkling with wisdom, kindness and a little mischief, and his laugh was positively infectious. The time passed so quickly and before we knew it, it was 1 a.m. and all the tubes had finished for the night. I had no idea how I was going to get back to Clapham.

'Well, I have my car,' Tom pointed out. 'I should be going too. I've got to be up early. Why don't I give you a lift? It's the least I can do after you bought me a drink.'

I accepted and so we left the party together, to raised eyebrows from Vivienne and Zoë (who told me later they had sat watching the two of us with amusement from across the room) and, still chatting, walked back to Tom's car. I had no idea where my house was in relation to where we were, so we consulted the London A–Z guide that Tom had in his car and headed off, around Hyde Park and through Kensington and Chelsea, past the Royal Court theatre and over Albert Bridge, the fascinating conversation continuing all the while. It took a long time to drive back to Clapham – ordinarily at 1 a.m. the journey should take about twenty minutes, but somehow it took us well over an hour. I was rather disappointed when we finally found my house.

'Well, we simply must keep in touch,' Tom said. 'I don't think I've ever had so much in common with someone. Ever.' He paused and smiled, as if letting that happy fact sink in for him. He typed my name – spelling it correctly without any prompting from me, another tick – and phone number into his phone and promised to be in touch soon. After a chaste but very charged kiss on the cheek, he drove away and I went inside. 'What a nice guy,' I smiled as I undressed and got into bed. 'I'll probably never see him again, but what a nice guy.'

*

'Soon' turned out to be the very next day. There was a friendly text (from him) followed by some Facebook stalking (from me), and then the dreamy smiles and butterflies in the stomach started. We sent each other excerpts from our writing projects and talked every day either via email or text until we finally met up again the following Saturday for dinner. This was the first date I had been excited about in a very long time. I wore a gorgeous floaty red dress from Washington DC that I couldn't really afford but hadn't been able to resist. While on the tube to Embankment station, I wrote on an Oscar Wilde postcard I'd found in a newsagent at the train station after work a few days earlier and decided to buy for Tom, to encourage him to 'keep looking at the stars' as we'd discussed that week. I wasn't sure whether this was coming across as too eager, as I had been with other men, but then I thought, *Stuff it. I would be so stoked if someone gave me something like this on the first date, so I'm just going to do it.* I was determined to be myself. I wasn't hiding any more. I liked who I was and if he didn't, I was confident I would be fine anyway.

I waited outside Embankment station for him and when he arrived, about fifteen minutes late as he'd forgotten the Victoria line was down on the weekends, he was even more handsome than I remembered. I now knew what chemistry felt like and as we walked across Jubilee Bridge to the South Bank I could feel it pulsing between us. We ate at Wagamama, a bustling canteen-style restaurant filled with Asian-inspired food, the air fragrant with garlic, chilli and coriander. We ate lovely food and the conversation looped through the threads of what we'd talked about the previous Saturday and over the week via email. It turned out Tom had lived in Melbourne for a time too. The conversation moved to our families and he told me some stories about his grandmother, who had died ten years earlier. I think I nearly choked on my mouthful of tofu fried rice. I remembered Nicole's words in Albuquerque of a few months earlier and felt both elated and terrified. *This wasn't part of the plan.*

After many hours, and when we had eaten the last bite of the wasabi chocolate cake we'd shared for dessert, we headed down along the South Bank for a slow, meandering walk in the warm, clear night, marvelling at how beautiful the city looked. We went into bookshops along the way and finally reached the Tate Modern and the Millennium Bridge. It was quite close to midnight by now and there was nothing else open, so we walked onto the bridge and stopped about halfway along to gaze at the beautiful city. St Paul's Cathedral was lit up in the moonlight and I could hear the Thames lapping below us. We leaned over the bridge and looked around, and then at each other. As St Paul's chimed midnight, we kept gazing shyly at each other and then he leaned in and kissed me, which was as wonderful as I had thought it would be, despite my being slightly paranoid that I had spring onion breath after all the Asian food (with no mints in my handbag). I half expected fireworks to erupt in the sky.

We walked up to Waterloo to catch a bus back to my place. I reached for his hand as we got to the end of the bridge, and the look on his face was priceless. 'None of my other girlfriends wanted to hold hands in public,' he admitted. 'They told me they thought it was too pukey.' I then became self-conscious of how I was holding his hand – with my thumb on top, which Dan had told me he didn't like while we were dating. I told Tom about that and he looked both shocked and amused. 'What a knob jockey,' he said, which made me laugh.

I gave him the Oscar Wilde postcard as we sat on the top level of the 59 bus to take us back to Brixton. I was embarrassed that the ink had smudged a little, but his reaction to this simple gesture on my part was very sweet. It was as if I had given him something precious. He certainly seemed very overwhelmed.

We had a cup of tea (not a euphemism) back at my place, and then he left after we made arrangements to see a piece of theatre in Camden Town the next evening. I went to bed straight away as it was incredibly late by then, but didn't sleep. I just lay there in a dazed state. The next morning, I grabbed the house phone and went back to bed with it, my international calling card and a cup of tea to ring my parents, which had become my Sunday morning routine.

'You've met someone,' Mum said as soon as she heard my voice.

'How can you tell?' I laughed.

'I just can. You sound happy.'

*

As Tom lived out of London at the time, but was coming up every weekend to work at the auction house, we spoke nearly every day and saw each other as often as we could on the days he was in the city. There was no suggestion he was growing tired of my company or needed (or preferred) to be somewhere else. Whenever he said he would call or come over, he (shock-horror) did! What a nice change. We still had the most fascinating conversations and every time we parted, I immediately started looking forward to seeing him again. It was as if I had known him my whole life. It was comfortable and yet so electrifying and exciting. Every time I saw him I thought I was going to burst and melt all at once.

One Friday night, when we'd only been seeing each other for a week or two, we met at the Tate Modern to see an exhibition, and then caught the tube and bus back to Battersea, where we had the flat to ourselves, as his sister was at a wedding in the country for the weekend. We cooked a meal together and as we made a salad and put potatoes on to boil, enjoying dreamy kisses in between tasks, I had a flashback to a few months earlier in Vancouver, when watching Sarah and Dave prepare dinner together had cemented everything I was looking and hoping for.

That night we revealed a great deal to each other – I told him that I was getting divorced, and he told me about some things that had happened to him that had changed him and set him on a very different path. As we finished eating and more wine was poured, we moved to the couch and he brought over a large book to show me. It was filled with cartoons and sketches, things he had drawn on his travels, notes, even a few short verses he'd penned. My heart leaped to my throat. *This wasn't part of the plan.*

I was trying very hard to live in the present, to enjoy it and not think too hard about where this might go. But the next morning as warm, happy light spilled through the windows and Tom brought me a cup of tea in bed, made exactly the way I liked it without him even having asked me, I knew it was only the beginning of something very, very special indeed.

You can't go home again

The weeks began to pass quickly and before too long my return to Australia for a family wedding (and ironically, to file for divorce myself) was merely days away. Things were still going incredibly well with Tom and every moment with him contained magical things I wanted to remember forever. I was completely unused to having someone want to share my activities and my life in such a meaningful way; to be making such an effort to see me and include me in his life and his plans. In the past it had always been me making the effort and, ultimately, the sacrifices. But I found it a little overwhelming because, as accurate as Nicole's predictions had proved so far, I began to worry I was only seeing what I wanted to see. I was determined not to be fooled again. While I knew in my heart that Tom was different, that his kindness and gentleness and our obvious love for each other was not put on and wouldn't be thrown back in my face at some later date when it was no longer convenient for him, there was a part of me that wouldn't allow me to believe it.

The reactions of a few people in my life to my new relationship did little to quell my fears that I perhaps didn't deserve this happiness and that I should be made to pay for my bad judgement and sinful divorce a little while longer. This cut quite deep because I expected that people who claimed to care for me, and for Tom too, would be happy for us but that was not always the case.

Vivienne was one of these people, to my huge disappointment. She had lived in London for over three years and hadn't yet met anyone she'd dated seriously. I had been there barely eight weeks and had met someone I suspected to be the love of my life so I guess it's understandable she was a bit resentful. At first she had been pleased that Tom and I had met through her, and felt I owed her one. But as the weeks went by and it was obvious that Tom and I were truly falling for each other, things turned a bit sour with Vivienne and never recovered. Every time she rolled her eyes at any mention of him, every time she referred to Tom and me as 'smug marrieds' and every time she reminded me I was still technically married to someone else, I winced a little. As with some of my other friends at this time, she had been so supportive when things were not going well for me but became quite a different person when things picked up. Why didn't I tell her where to go, I hear you ask? Well, it was tricky because she was subtle with her putdowns and by the time I realised what she'd said, the moment was over. Her snippy pinpricks and jealous remarks continued, as did my excuses for them, and eventually we simply lost touch.

At this time I had also started to hear rumours of some unflattering things being said about me by some bloggers back in Australia. A reader from Sydney, someone I had never even met, emailed me. 'I'm so sorry to do this,' she wrote, 'but you seem to be such a nice, genuine person and I think you deserve to know what these people are saying about you.'

It turned out a blogger who I'll call Mel, who lived in Sydney but spent a lot of time in Melbourne, had begun what can only be described as a character assassination of me, roping in as many members of the blogging community as she could – including some women in Melbourne I had thought of as good friends, like Gillian. I'd only met Mel a handful of times and while I thought she was a little strange and clearly had a few issues, for the most part she had been extremely friendly and supportive, to my face. Now, Mel had started a smear campaign against me with the ruthlessness of a tabloid newspaper, particularly with regard to my personal life after the separation. She had even dragged Glenn into her spiteful judgements, despite having never met him. Everything I'd ever written on my blog was a pack of lies, according to her. She had the *real* scoop on Skinny Latte. She had twisted some things I had said – things I had mostly said to take the piss (out of myself) or where I was merely thinking aloud (not smart, I now realise) – and initiated many gossiping sessions with Melbourne bloggers in which I was the main topic of conversation. At least that explained why Gillian had dropped off the face of the earth: she had been feeding Mel's fire. Apparently both women had recently written blog posts that were thinly veiled attacks on me, but when I went to read them for myself I found I had been blocked.

The best part of a decade later, I can see it all for the storm in a teacup it was, but it was my first real taste of bullying in my adult life and frankly it reminded me of school, where I had been a nice girl and hence an easy target. But this wasn't a handful of bitchy girls in a suburb of Hobart; this character assassination had crossed state lines and gone international. The fact that Mel was still being chummy to me added to my disgust and confusion – she'd even emailed me to say she was going to be in London soon and wanted to catch up! Even though what she, and others, were doing was unfair, cruel and hurtful, I felt I didn't really have any recourse other than to confront them, and we all know how good I was at that. I think I thought if I just ignored them they would eventually get bored and leave me alone. But as anyone who has ever been bullied will tell you, ignoring it rarely achieves anything.

I had been incredibly naive, looking back. While the friendships I had made through my blog had for the most part been overwhelmingly wonderful, I had never once considered that a bunch of women blogging about weight loss were bound to have some emotional problems. But as I had been working on my issues and taking ownership for my shit, I had assumed they were too. I thought we were all in this together. But we weren't, as it turned out. I wasn't one of them any more. The women behind this malevolence had lost and gained the same five or ten kilograms over the period I had known them, whereas I had been at my goal weight for coming up to two years. It didn't take a genius to figure out what their problem with me was.

Despite this, I was gutted. I had felt valued and accepted for who I was for the first time in my adult life among these people. They had rejoiced in my success with my weight loss, and had been so supportive through my separation and newfound single freedom. To find out that some of them had now turned on me like this, and that I had been so deceived in their regard for me, was devastating.

But something that cuts even deeper than noise from your enemies is the silence of a friend. In that respect, the worst was yet to come.

*

I was sad to be leaving Tom for a month when we were still in this new and fresh phase of our relationship, and when I had just started to feel at home in London. He had started being slightly distant with me, which had made me a bit paranoid. He told me later it was merely a self-preservation thing – this was exactly how his other Australian girlfriend had left the UK, leaving a few things at his place with the promise that she would be back within a certain period of time. Instead, it was a year before he saw her again and by that time she'd decided they were 'just friends'. I can now see why he was wary. To make matters worse, I was departing on Tom's birthday – a date I had plucked out of thin air at the STA office at Melbourne University many months earlier.

'Just come back, darling,' were Tom's final words when we said goodbye at Heathrow. 'That's all I ask.'

On my way back to Australia, I stopped in Copenhagen and Singapore, the remaining cities on my round-the-world ticket, and stayed with a lovely blog reader in each place. I was still overwhelmed by the generosity of people who knew me but had never met me and by the incredibly wide reach of my little blog, though I hadn't updated it all that much these days. I thoroughly enjoyed staying with these kind people and seeing their adopted cities – they too were expats – through their eyes, adding more stamps to a passport that had been empty the year before.

I landed in Perth and within days of being back in Australia, things started to unravel. I was exhausted, jet-lagged and running a bit of a fever after going from sub-zero Copenhagen to tropical Singapore to dry and dusty Perth within a week. I was also feeling heartsick at being apart from Tom. I missed him terribly and my general tiredness from travelling had done nothing for my paranoia. Despite having been so confident and happy when I left London, I was convinced that now I was out of sight, I was definitely going to be out of mind. I tortured myself with these thoughts day and night. One of my biggest triggers for anxiety is tiredness. I can't think straight and can't talk myself out of a loop of crazy thinking. I take things personally on a good night's sleep; when I'm tired I'm the Olympic champion of sensitivity. The difference is now I make myself a cup of tea, read a book and go to bed. But back then, I either didn't recognise the triggers or ignored them. I pushed on. The wise, reassuring person I thought I had become was nowhere to be seen.

I had been in Perth about two days. One morning, I eventually stumbled downstairs, still jet-lagged but feeling reasonably well rested. Brenda, the blogging friend I had once hosted in Melbourne and who was now returning the favour, saw me come down the stairs and came over and gave me a hug, a sad look on her face. Confused, I braced myself for some terrible news.

'Someone's left a really horrible comment on your blog,' she said sombrely, delivered in the same tone as 'There's been an accident.' I read the comment. It had been left anonymously but the commenter was pretending to be my parents, saying how ashamed they were of me. It made reference to anything sexual I had ever mentioned on the blog – namely two posts in which I had talked about being single again and getting the Brazilian wax, both of them from well over a year ago. The comment ended with my parents' email address – their correct one – as if to give the anonymous vitriol the stamp of authenticity.

I'm embarrassed at how quickly I forgot everything I'd learned with Jules and went back to acting like a frightened bullied teenager. If it happened now, I would just laugh because it was so ridiculous, then delete it and get on with my day. But at that moment in time, that wasn't going to happen. I was completely stunned that someone would be so nasty. Meredith was suddenly on the phone. It was she who had alerted Brenda to the comment in the first place – they had been discussing it while I was asleep. The troll's identity was a mystery, and one that Brenda and Meredith were determined to focus on. I didn't know if it was remnants of jet-lag or the shock of such a bizarre personal attack but I was shaking. I put my head in my hands. What a mess. I just wanted to be left alone. Maybe continuing to share aspects of my life in a public medium that left me open to exposure and attacks like this was a bad idea. As much as the blog had enriched my life beyond anything I could have imagined, especially when I lived in Melbourne and on my travels, I had moved well beyond my reasons for starting it and maybe this, together with the general nastiness aimed in my direction lately, was a huge sign I should just delete the whole thing. I said as much to Meredith and Brenda.

I could be wrong, as it was a long time ago now, but I don't recall either of them offering reassurance that this anonymous commenter was just some complete loser with nothing better to do, and that the best thing I could do was delete the comment and move on; that taking the blog down would be letting this bully, whoever they were, win. They just seemed highly intrigued by the drama, trying to figure out who in the blogging community had the biggest axe to grind with me. Meredith let slip that Mel and Gillian were definitely still on the warpath, so that upset me even more.

Emotional, frightened and fed up, I decided to delete the blog. This wasn't what I'd signed up for. I was tired of the popularity contest this previously very supportive and caring online community had become. It was too much like high school now. I wanted no part of it. I would leave it to the bullies and the trolls.

I deleted the mean comment and wrote a quick farewell post, with Meredith and Brenda's encouragement, but almost the minute the post went live, the nastiness started again. 'Are you doing this because of the comment left by your parents?' snarked Anonymous. They had clearly been waiting for my reaction. But there were some very kind comments too and they well and truly crowded out the nasty ones, which I discovered later were all left by the same person pretending to be three or four different people ganging up on me. To my surprise, even Glenn weighed in with a pleasant comment, which led Meredith and Brenda to say some unflattering things about him, even though Meredith had only met him a handful of times and Brenda had never met him at all. It became clear that I, and the details of my life, had been a popular topic of conversation for these people for some time.

After a few hours, when I felt the farewell post had been up long enough, I pressed the delete button and Skinny Latte, my beloved blog, was no more, just a memory and an invalid URL. I remember sitting there on Brenda's couch, feeling strange, like I'd lost something I wasn't quite ready to let go of just yet. Something I should have fought harder for.

*

I was relieved to leave Perth and land in Hobart. Mum, my sister Rebekah and my nearly four-year-old nephew were there to meet me. The latter two raced over to me and flew into my arms, as if I had never left. I inhaled deeply as we all walked out to the car – that beautiful fresh Hobart air, pure oxygen, sweet with the smell of gum trees. I hadn't realised how much I'd missed it.

Several days later, an express post envelope arrived for me at Mum and Dad's. It was the divorce papers, filled in and signed by Glenn. It had all been relatively straightforward. We had spoken on the phone for the first time in over a year, which had been very awkward to start with but once I'd allowed Glenn to boast about how well he was doing, the conversation moved on to other things and, despite the superficial nature of it, I could tell he had grown up a little. He had moved on. I could finally see that his annoying and immature behaviour in the aftermath of the separation had happened because he was in pain and I was the only person he could take it out on.

We amicably discussed the details of how we would go about finalising the divorce. Glenn would get the forms, fill in his sections, get his part witnessed and send them down to me in Hobart, with

244

a cheque for his share of the court fees. I would then fill in my part and file the documents. It sounded easy.

While I was relieved to eventually hang up the phone, I also felt happy. Happy we had been able to wish each other well, happy we both now wanted all this official stuff taken care of so it would be well and truly over.

I scanned the papers that had arrived, filled in with the details we'd agreed on. There was also a small photo attached to the first page of the legal documents with a tiny paper clip. I recognised it as the photo of me as a child Glenn used to keep in his wallet. I must have been three years old when it was taken; playing on the beach, my blonde hair cut pixie-short, flashing a smile filled with milky baby teeth. There was no note, nothing. Just this photo.

That same day I headed down to the Commonwealth law courts in Davey Street, expecting there to be a big scary sign saying 'Divorces this way', but it turned out to be like going to any other government service centre, like getting a Medicare refund or your car registration sorted out. I was the only person there. A friendly-looking woman called me over to the desk and took a thorough look through my papers.

'This all seems straightforward,' she said, clicking her tongue as she turned the pages. 'Yes, it's been more than a year since you separated ... no dependents ... easy. This will take five minutes.' She typed merrily into a computer, stopping briefly to ask me for the marriage certificate, which I handed over. One of her colleagues came over to ask her something. 'Just a sec, I'm just doing a divorce for this lady,' she said breezily.

I almost laughed at the casualness of it, as if this woman

processed this kind of thing every day – which, I realised, she probably did.

'Right, the next hearing I can get you into is the thirtieth,' the woman explained once she had entered all the details. 'Because it's so straightforward you don't need to be there and it should go through absolutely fine. Once the divorce is granted, it becomes final one month and one day from November thirtieth.'

'New Year's Eve.' I said, thinking aloud.

The woman laughed. 'Two reasons to celebrate then!'

'And what happens during that one month and one day?'

'Well, either of you can change your mind during that time. But on December thirty-first, it's final. That's it. You'll get some documents sent to your registered address. The decree nisi, it's called. Keep it safe. You'll need it if you get married again.'

I paid the fee and the woman stamped a few more documents and handed them over to me. She smiled. 'Congratulations. Good luck.'

I had been waiting for what felt like years for that moment, when it would all be officially over. I went outside, the November sky now filled with grey clouds. To my surprise, Mum was at the bottom of the courthouse steps, her floral scarf fluttering in the breeze, waiting for me. She wrapped me in a warm hug. 'I thought we should go and celebrate,' she said, smiling.

We walked down the road to Salamanca Square, where we went into a bar and got two glasses of Jansz sparkling, which were as bright as Mum's eyes as she looked over at me.

'How do you feel?' she asked.

I felt deeply relieved but, oddly enough, also a bit hollow. This was another ending, and there had been so many of them in my life recently. Ever since that horrible night the year before I'd tried so hard to start living the life I'd always wanted to live but it really hadn't been easy. I'd made so many mistakes and, from what I could tell, I'd been judged harshly for them by some people. And now I had Tom, this wonderful man who I knew I wanted to be with, but I hadn't seen him for nearly a month and was feeling fragile and insecure about that. Why was I feeling so down? When was my bright new beginning going to happen?

Mum smiled gently and squeezed my hand. 'Phil,' she said, 'this *is* your bright new beginning. I know this isn't exactly what you thought your life would look like, but you have nothing to be ashamed of. It all needed to happen so you would become who you needed to be.'

'Oh, Mum.' I sighed tearfully.

Mum picked up the glasses and handed me one. We clinked them gently. 'Here's to a brand new start for you,' Mum said. And we drank to that.

*

Before I knew it, it was time to go to Melbourne for a few days and await my flight back to London. I had booked a one-way ticket back, which had pretty much emptied my savings account, but I knew that was where I wanted to be. I had loved being back in Hobart, in the loving embrace of my family, where I felt relaxed and safe. Melbourne was different. Several friends there had grown distant in the six months I'd been gone and didn't respond to my messages. Angela hadn't spoken to me since she had cancelled her trip to London.

While I was overwhelmed with nostalgia and love for Melbourne as I wandered its streets again, I was also glad I didn't live there any more as there were a lot of sad memories. Having said that, being back in Melbourne reaffirmed some of my greatest friendships, with people whose company truly made my heart sing. I had wonderful times with Ashley, Ming-Zhu, Louise and even some old colleagues. Mary and Daniel flew down from Sydney especially to see me, which was wonderful.

I hadn't been sleeping well since Perth. I was taking medication to sleep, as my anxious mind was constantly going over of all the nastiness, doubt and disappointments. It was made much worse by my arrival in Melbourne. Meredith was there to meet me at the airport and I had actually been really looking forward to seeing her. She had been very supportive since I shut down my blog. It was as if the awkwardness between us during my last few months in Australia had been resolved at last. She had the day off work and we drove straight to Daylesford, a town about two hours out of Melbourne, to recreate a happy day we had once spent there together.

The first time we'd gone it had been September the year before, just as I had broken up with James. Meredith had wanted to cheer me up. Spring hadn't yet arrived and it was still freezing cold. Nothing was growing; the trees were bare and pinecones rotted whole into the earth. We went for a massage at one of the spas in the springs, and my masseur had a broken fingernail that scratched me. I felt I couldn't ask him to do anything about it. It just made me want to cry. But eating lavender scones, wandering the quaint shops and markets and walking through the acres of dormant lavender bushes, still fragrant with the promise of a flowering summer, made me feel better. Meredith and I talked a lot that day, about many things, and I felt very close to her. We played favourite songs from our high school years in the car and sang along at the top of our lungs, and ate so many peanut M&Ms I had to undo the top button of my jeans on the drive home.

This time, the November heat was suffocating. The heaviness in the air intensified the lavender's fragrance: heady, all pervading. We drank iced ginger mint tea to quash the burn of heat in our throats. The lavender scones came, buried in avalanches of cream, and I ate greedily, the sweetness momentarily numbing the emptiness inside, a coping mechanism I remembered well.

It was harder to be with Meredith this time. She tearfully confessed that not only had she known, all year, about the nasty and vindictive behaviour of Mel and Gillian (it had started while I was still living in Melbourne, apparently) but that she had joined in. When she told me that, all of a sudden her behaviour at the start of the year made complete sense. She had eventually withdrawn from it, and told these women she didn't want to be dragged into bitchy conversations about me any more, but unlike the sympathetic reader in Sydney, she didn't think I deserved to be defended or to be made aware of what had been happening. Her reason for all of this? 'I was really unhappy at the time.'

As if this wasn't hard enough to hear, she made this confession at a time and place where it was impossible for me to get angry with her. If I made a scene and stormed off, I would be the one making the huge drama. I would be the one who ruined our lovely day out. Not to mention the fact I would be stranded two hours out of Melbourne. I felt like she had deliberately orchestrated it so she could unload her burden of guilt in such a way that I would just have to let it go.

I know I could have, and should have, handled the situation differently but I was a fragile mess who just wanted to go back to England, fall into the arms of the man I loved and get on with my life. It also occurred to me to wonder, if this was how Meredith had behaved behind my back when we were supposedly friends, what she would do if I got angry and told her where to go. So I put on a brave face and tried to carry on. I thought I was protecting myself but in actual fact I was holding at arm's length all the discomfort I didn't want to feel. Those three days in Melbourne, staying with her and Justin, were horrible, even though Meredith was being very sweet and acting as though nothing had happened. I should have just gone to a hotel; I don't really know why I didn't. The whole time I stayed with them I had nightmares that had me waking up in tears. I felt so broken.

When I finally got back to London, I planned to give Meredith a wide berth and hope she'd get the hint. Instead, I got a lot of 'You've been really quiet lately, hope nothing's wrong' emails, which just made me feel guilty. But within that guilt there was a core of anger. Anger that she had betrayed me; that so many of my happy memories of Melbourne were now tainted; that she felt even remotely justified in her behaviour; and that I had been so deceived.

It wasn't safe for me to shine – that was the message I received from the whole ordeal. Being myself – my abundant, shiny, crazy self – and being proud of all I had achieved was not okay, and suddenly felt frightening for the first time since all this change had begun. People had got so nasty. It seemed to confirm my greatest fear – I was being myself, and putting my own happiness first, and I had been rejected. I had to press the mute button. Again.

Not only was I furious at these women, I was bitterly disappointed in them too. Why do women attack each other like this? Why is it so hard to be happy when other people, your friends no less, succeed? Life isn't easy, for any of us. We should be better than this. I didn't know why being happy, confident and proud of yourself was interpreted as 'swapping a big body for a big ego', as Meredith actually put it at one point.

I've caught myself pausing as I wrote about these events. I wonder whether any of those women will read this book. I'm sure they would remember all of this very differently – but perhaps they wouldn't. Looking back I can see how desperately unhappy they all were. We had all been in the same boat once, but I'd jumped out and started swimming. As such, they saw me as a threat and cast me out. Perhaps they found the changes I'd been brave enough to make too confronting. Maybe it was easier to demonise me than it was for them to dig deep and face their own demons. Maybe they felt I now had far too high an opinion of myself and needed taking down a few pegs. Maybe they were simply jealous. Who knows? What I do know is theirs were not the actions of happy people content with their lives. The hate they directed at me was only a reflection of how much they hated themselves.

The biggest mistake I made at this time was not sharing any of it with Tom. I hadn't even really told him about the blog. He told me years later that he knew something was up. 'The girl who left the UK in October and the girl who came back in November were two very different people,' he said. 'It was like a light had gone out in you. You looked so scared when you came out into arrivals at Heathrow. It was like you didn't believe I would be there.' That was the truth. Having been whacked by one emotional sledgehammer after another in the month I'd been gone, I was fully expecting to find Tom had changed his mind about me too. I was convinced everyone was out to get me, conveniently forgetting that the nastiness had only really come from a handful of people. I was wounded and hurt, so the bullies got exactly what they wanted. I disappeared.

My brave face was still the mask I wore every day. I told myself the best revenge was having a happy life so I was determined to make a success of myself in London and keep writing and striving. My divorce went through without a hitch, and Tom and I saw in 2008 together with wine, fireworks and hopeful plans of what the year would hold for us. I was free. I was living in the most magnificent city in the world. I was young, I had the world at my feet, I had a gorgeous man who I loved and who loved me.

Everything should now be perfect.

Right?

PART THREE

Chai Latte

'There are only two ways to live –
as a victim or as a courageous fighter.'

NIKKI GEMMELL, *HONESTLY*

Striking back

The following year, 2008, was a strange year. Everything felt unfamiliar as I settled into real life in a new country. Not only that but all my baggage had come with me, and not just the kind with luggage labels. By returning to Australia at the end of the year before, I'd had to face everything I'd wanted to leave behind and forget. Without the blog, which I hadn't realised I'd come to rely on for my self-confidence in the past two years, I was floundering. I had become so dependent on it for validation, for acceptance, for feeling good about myself, that I had lost the ability to feel worthy without it.

All my journal entries from that year fall into three categories: rage-filled outbursts of the hurt and pain I was carrying around, trying to find my confidence again as if it were merely a pair of sunglasses I'd left in a bar; notes and ideas for writing projects and subsequent lambasting of myself when those projects didn't go anywhere; and love-filled, dreamy musings about Tom and our growing relationship.

I'll come back to the first two, but in terms of my new love, things couldn't have been going better. Tom got a new job in London and needed to move to the city; I was unhappy in my lodgings, so we decided we would live together. After a bit of searching, we ended up in a two-bedroom flat in Southgate, in London's north. We had only been together about eight months so it was a little fast, perhaps, but I was so excited. I loved everything about him – his passion, his grace and courage, his sense of humour, the way he saw the world, how freely and without condition he had given me his heart. Living together was everything I hoped it would be and everything my previous experience of living with a partner hadn't been. Even six months in, we still looked at each other with a bit of excited disbelief in the mornings when we woke up to realise the other was there, and exchanging kisses or a cheeky smile over the boiling kettle as we made tea, as if to say, 'Can you believe this? We live together!' We were so happy to see each other when we came home every day. Sometimes we would even end up in the same carriage on the same Piccadilly line tube home. If you've ever caught a tube in London at peak hour, you'll know how unlikely that is. And not only was I thrilled my boyfriend was vegetarian too, it was also wonderful to have someone to cook and plan meals for again. Tom was incredibly appreciative and complimentary of my cooking – perhaps he was just grateful not to be living off the typical British bachelor fare of boil-in-the-bag curries or baked beans on toast any more. He often commented that he had never eaten so many green vegetables in his life.

It took a little getting used to though, as my living arrangements had been haphazard for the last two years to say the least, and I had become accustomed to only having myself to consider. Tom was the same. He had lived alone for over five years and enjoyed playing Nine Inch Nails at full blast and staying up until 2 a.m. watching films or writing. He had never lived with a girlfriend before, so it was all new territory for him. It was fun and cute, as we got used to each other and our various habits, but it wasn't without its challenges. Our first trip to IKEA together was certainly interesting! It was towards the end of 2008 that I began to realise, despite how happy we were together, how low my self-worth had sunk, and how it was starting to affect Tom as well. That wasn't good. It was then I realised I needed help again.

It took a long time for me to admit that though – that I had stopped being the heroine of my life and somehow ended up a victim again. I had forgotten that being the heroine (or hero) of your own life is hard work. It requires consistent effort on your part; you have to believe in yourself and you have to work on it every single day. You have to be relentless in your search for the positive, which isn't easy. Being the victim, on the other hand, is. A few days of feeling sorry for yourself very easily stretches into a month, then that month becomes a year. If you don't realise this is what you're doing and get in the driver's seat again, then before you know it, being the victim is your only story.

How did it happen to me? I was utterly deflated after the events of the end of 2007, devastated by the betrayal of my so-called friends,

frightened to ever put myself out into the arena again, much as I
yearned to be there. Instead of being proud of my weight-loss success and of the fact I'd survived a divorce and come out the other
side willing to take a chance on love again, I was now deeply ashamed
of all of it. I was terrified that my voice would be ridiculed and
judged and torn apart. I was so wrapped up in my hurt and how
unfair it had all been to see that responding this way was indeed a
choice. And as for everything else, well, I thought I'd already worked
hard enough, that the days of having to put in a constant rigorous
effort to stay on top of my issues were over and I could relax. I
thought that with all I had been through and survived, the rest of
my life would be easy.

I do want to shake 2008 Phil a bit, I'll be honest. Why couldn't
I see it? Like my mother had said, this *was* my new beginning. I
just hadn't expected it to be like this. But living a life you're proud
of is not easy. Living authentically and consciously is not easy.
Going after your dreams is not easy. If any of it were, everyone
would do it.

I could go on for pages about how discouraged and unhappy I
was in 2008. But perhaps it's more productive if I tell you what I
learned.

I learned that if you aren't happy with who you are, the size on
your clothing tags or being able to run 10 kilometres without stopping really doesn't matter. Both shopping and exercise are more
enjoyable when you love your body, not when you use those activities to punish yourself.

I learned that moving to a new country comes with a lengthy
settling-in period, and when the awesomeness of it all wears off the

blues can set in, when you just want *something* to be familiar, and after one too many 'Sorry, you need to be a citizen to do that' conversations. This is normal and to be expected. You can't take any of it personally.

I learned that it's very hard on your partner when you don't love yourself. It turns you into a needy, clingy person and whatever love they give you will never be enough. If you believe, on any level, that you do not deserve to be loved, you will only (albeit unconsciously) punish those who try.

I learned that there's no trick to being self-confident. You simply accept that you are okay, just as you are, even if nobody is saying or doing anything to reassure you of that fact.

I learned that not everyone you lose from your life is a loss. If there are people in your life whose company flattens rather than uplifts you, you need to address that rather than shy away from confrontation. You're allowed to stand up for yourself. Try it. I wish I had.

I learned you have to find ways to be resilient in life. We need the good stuff in our lives, but we also need to be able to pick ourselves up, not only when we fall but when we are deliberately tripped.

I learned that if you haven't got your mental health, you don't really have much at all.

*

When 2008 finally turned into 2009, I resolved that this was the year I would get myself back on track. I had spent the past year feeling defeatist, paranoid and insecure, questioning everything good in my life because so many things I'd believed were good – mostly friendships – had fallen apart. And even if I did find happiness and success again, I was convinced someone would find a way of ruining it for me. It was exhausting, for me and the people around me. I was determined to sort this out. Otherwise, what had been the point of it all? Had I really learned nothing over the past four years? I couldn't do it on my own though, that much was obvious. I'd struggled through 2008 trying to prop myself up, and I'd sometimes be okay for a few days but then something would happen and I'd spiral down again. I just couldn't deal rationally with life's little knocks any more. I needed another Jules.

On a rainy Wednesday night in January after work, I took the tube out to Liverpool Street and wandered the dark, freezing alleyways to meet my new counsellor. I felt a good rapport with Margot straight away – very important if you're going to do the work you need to do. She was like a really cool auntie, the type who would teach you to swear or play poker, someone who was totally on my side but wasn't afraid to give me some tough love either.

She said I deserved to feel very proud of how far I'd come. 'I can't wait to see what you do next,' she said, smiling. She also said all the issues I had come to her with – feeling low, betrayed, paranoid and inadequate; fear of missing out; and feeling guilty for being a success – all stemmed back to deeper, more painful experiences. If I acknowledged and dealt with those, then perhaps I'd be able to move on from the events of the past year.

In the year that I visited Margot every week, she taught me a great deal, especially how to handle my anxieties, paranoia and negative thinking. I realised I was sticking to old beliefs about myself and should be embracing the good things about my life now instead of believing it was all some kind of fluke that would be taken away. I also realised that I had fought hard for the happiness and confidence I had felt prior to the end of 2007. If I wanted that again, I had to fight for it again.

'You've still got quite a bit of growing up to do, sweetie,' Margot said on more than one occasion. 'Life isn't fair. You've got to work hard for everything. Even if you've already worked hard. And you can't expect things to change if all you're doing is sitting around feeling sorry for yourself.'

Margot encouraged me to be more proactive in my life, to make things happen for myself rather than waiting for permission. I hadn't waited for permission to lose weight and get fit, had I? I had to apply that determination to every other area of my life, especially my writing. I was working hard at it and feeling frustrated about not having my work out in the world any more, but a part of me was also working hard to keep me small. I was terrified if I dared to shine again, as brightly as I wanted to and knew I could, I was asking for the nastiness of 2007 to recur. I had internalised it, as I had when I had been bullied at school, and made it my fault, something that had been in my control, which of course it hadn't been. It took a long time for my thinking to change on that.

Margot also told me at some point, when the opportunity arose, I would need to confront the people who were still in my life who had hurt me, namely Meredith. This was tricky because to avoid receiving plaintive 'You're being quiet, hope nothing's wrong' emails, I still kept in touch with her, giving her no reason to think her betrayal had devastated me as much as it had. Trying to repair the friendship would have been hard enough if we'd been in the same city; being on the other side of the world made it damn near impossible. I knew telling her the truth would hurt her, which I didn't want to do, despite everything. But slowly I realised that if on the other side of that was freedom from the heaviness of taking on someone else's guilt, it simply had to be done.

I also began to realise I wasn't alone. The last few years of my life had been all about big changes and dramatic transformations. Now it had become something else; it had settled down, and I now just had to focus on maintaining both my weight and my new life. My friend, the writer Shauna Reid, put it perfectly: 'Maintenance isn't all that different to weight loss. Some days it's fabulous. Some days it sucks. And that's okay.' I remembered there were other people out there who understood and I could reach out and let them in. I just had to be more careful this time.

As a result, 2009 was the year I started blogging again. I felt my interest in health and fitness return as the fog began to lift and my confidence slowly resurfaced. I also noticed some of my blogging buddies back in Australia who hadn't gone to the dark side in 2007 were hitting a few roadblocks with their own journeys and I wanted to be a support for them again. I wanted them to be reminded of how well we had done together, back in the 'old days', and that we could do it again.

Weight-loss statistics are depressing – it's estimated 95 per cent of people who lose weight will gain it back again. It has taken me years to realise that I did too – not the physical weight, but all the emotional kilograms were stacked back on after the events of 2007 and 2008. After thinking that lonely and insecure young woman I used to be was dead and buried, I realised she had actually been there the whole time and I had been keeping her quiet, just not with food. I needed to deal with her again. I needed reminding that the reason I succeeded with my weight loss in the first place was because I was so upbeat and motivated; I believed in myself and always looked for the silver lining, even when the scales said the same weight four weeks in a row. I had to get back in the same headspace to get my mental health back. Just as I had had to learn new habits like going for a walk or a run every day after work, eating more vegetables and less ice-cream, I also had to learn new emotional habits like checking in with my feelings, paying attention, making the time to treat myself well and standing up for myself. I thought I had learned these things already but I clearly hadn't. Perhaps everything from 2006 to now had been one long distraction, keeping me from doing the permanent habit-building that I needed to do.

The response to the reappearance of Skinny Latte in the blogosphere with her second incarnation – Skinny Latte Strikes Back – was nothing short of humbling. The more posts I wrote, the more I realised how much I had learned from losing weight. It had been a doorway into what else was possible in my life. I couldn't believe how easily I had forgotten that anything I was not 100 per cent happy with in my life could be changed, with hard work, dedication and a positive attitude. It was never too late to start again. I felt stronger every day, knowing that sharing my struggles was helping others. The worst thing I did in 2008 was hide away, keeping my shame alive, and the best thing I did in 2009 was come back out of the shadows.

*

Life in London continued to delight. Tom and I moved to a new flat in April that year, to a central area called Pimlico, very close to Victoria station, the Thames embankment and Westminster Abbey. The tiny one-bedroom basement flat with a courtyard garden was a bit dilapidated and grotty, and the bathroom and kitchen were barely big enough for the two of us to be in at the same time, but we were charmed by the area. We could both walk to work instead of taking a crowded tube every day. Battersea Park was only a mile in one direction, St James's Park a mile in the other. The magnificent art gallery Tate Britain was merely a few minutes' walk away. There were pubs, coffee shops and even a library on our street. We could hear Big Ben striking the hour when we sat in the living room. We didn't have much money but because the financial crisis had started to hit Britain hard, rents were actually reasonable for possibly the first time in history. We still don't know how we managed to score a bargain flat in such a great central area, but for the two and a half years we spent in Pimlico, we soaked up as much of our beloved city as we possibly could.

In October 2009, Tom and I went to Australia together for the first time to attend another family wedding. This was the first time most of my family and friends would meet him, so even though we'd been together for over two years by then, it was still a little daunting for him. He had of course met them all over Skype and my parents had paid us a visit in the summer the year before, and so had various relatives and friends who had transited through London, so I had no concerns. I was particularly excited for him to meet my sisters, who I knew would love him.

The trip had a slight cloud over it, as my grandmother passed away just before we flew back. We had always been very close and I know how much she would have adored Tom. She had been unwell for some time and had recently gone to live in a nursing home. I got a phone call from Mum one morning as I was leaving for work to tell me Nan had had a fall at the home, broken her hip and was now in hospital. The prognosis wasn't great, given her increasing frailty and poor health of late, and she hadn't regained consciousness since the fall. A day or two passed and there had been no change. She was still hanging on. 'I think she's waiting for you,' Mum said.

Our flight to Hobart was ten days away. The idea of Nan lying there, in pain, until I got there was heartbreaking. Her life had been far from easy, having lived with profound deafness since childhood and beaten breast cancer not once, but four times. I didn't want her to suffer any more.

At about midnight I got into bed and looked over at the framed photo I had of Nan on my dressing table.

'I love you, Nan,' I said. 'Don't worry about me, I'll be fine. Don't wait for me to come home. If you need to go now, I understand. Just go. I'll be all right.'

Tom came in from brushing his teeth, we turned out the light and went to sleep. Twenty minutes later, the phone rang. It was my father, with the sad news that Nan had gone.

'When?' I asked, assuming it had been hours ago and they were only just getting around to telling me.

'About twenty minutes ago,' Dad said.

I lay there for a while, abandoning the idea of sleep. While I was heartbroken she was gone, I felt I had been able to say goodbye in some way, and I was glad the last time I saw Nan she was the same feisty and lively woman she had always been. Funnily enough, even though she couldn't physically hear me, I felt like she was the one person in my life who would always listen. What happened that night proved that beyond any doubt. I miss her still.

Apart from the grief and the strangeness of being home without Nan there, our return to Hobart was glorious. The trip was just what I was hoping for. Lots of quality time with people I loved, reconnecting, exploring, sharing. It was wonderful to show Tom around my hometown and take him to all my favourite places, to introduce him to people he'd heard me talk about for the past two years, to show him where I'd come from.

Towards the end of the trip, Tom revealed he had asked my parents' permission to propose to me. I thought I was going to pass out with happiness when he told me that. Until that moment, I hadn't realised how much I wanted to marry him. Every time that thought had popped into my head over the last two years, I'd flicked it away like an annoying insect. Bizarrely, my past experience hadn't completely put me off marriage. I think I was just terrified of making the same mistake, of being caught off guard and it all going wrong again. The idea of ever being divorced again overwhelmed me with shame, but the only way I could guarantee it would never happen was if I never married again. And the idea of not being married to this wonderful man was unthinkable. I had never known love like this. We adored each other yet didn't put each other on a pedestal. We felt safe with each other. We accepted each other, for all our strengths and weaknesses. He was thoughtful, generous, gentle and brave – everything I had ever wanted. Our relationship wasn't perfect but that was actually what made it so.

I'd talked to my father about it while I was home. 'How will I know if I'm ready for this again?' I asked him.

'You won't,' he said simply. 'You'll just have to take a leap of faith and trust what you have.'

*

I was sorry to leave Hobart but excited about a few days in Melbourne with our wonderful friends Ming-Zhu and Nicholas, who were also to be married soon (but we sadly couldn't stick around long enough for their wedding), and with Ashley, John and their little family. An old friend even flew down from Brisbane especially to see us. My spirit was renewed and inspired by my friends' company and by how much they loved Tom and welcomed him. While there were still a few ghosts in Melbourne, they weren't howling as loudly as the last time. I loved being there with Tom. We both had different memories of living there and it was wonderful to make new ones.

As expected, I didn't hear from Meredith until after we left, even though she knew when we'd be in town. I hadn't planned to go out of my way to see her – if she got in touch, I would have happily met up but would have had a few things to say, none of which she would have felt comfortable hearing. I think she knew that, which was why I hadn't, to my great relief, heard much from her in the last few months. The thing was, I had forgiven her for what she'd done – I just didn't want her in my life any more. But in Singapore, while I was killing time between flights and making use of free airport wi-fi, there was her name in my inbox. She said she felt 'weird' having to chase me, but it was obvious I was back in Australia and she was disappointed I hadn't made arrangements to see her. 'I hope I haven't done anything to upset you?' was how she signed it off. I couldn't believe it.

I sent a short message back, explaining that the visit had been very busy and I hadn't had time to chase anyone, but that she knew when I would be in the country and I would have been perfectly happy to see her if she'd had the guts to face me. If it was too 'weird' for her to contact me, that was her problem. What had she been expecting, given what she had put me through last time? It was blunt and to the point, very unlike me, but I felt I couldn't leave any room for ambiguity this time. I held my breath as I hit send.

Meredith responded almost immediately, with a very, very long email wherein all my failings throughout our friendship were discussed in great detail, which suggested she had been expecting this. She had put up with so much from me, she said. Being taken for granted, hot and cold manipulative behaviour, exclusion from other parts of my social life. I had apparently made her feel more worthless than she had ever felt in her entire life. On and on it went. *Is this a friend talking or an ex-lover?* I wondered, confused and alarmed by the intensity of it.

She admitted that she had wanted to 'rescue' me in the immediate aftermath of my separation. Seeing me, the girl who'd reached her goal and supposedly had it all, fall from grace, as it were, she had wanted to be the person who got me through it. She wanted me to need her. And when I didn't 'need' her in the same way any more, she had taken that very badly, which was why she had gone on to do what she did. And if I was still angry about her betrayal then fine, but why had I strung her along, pretending everything was okay?

I did feel bad about that. But at the same time, if I had indeed been such a terrible friend, why had she wanted to see me at all?

I had my answer when she mentioned her great embarrassment that she'd had to fend off interrogation from the blogging community about whether she had seen me. I suspected all along that her indignation at being slighted did not come from a genuine desire to see me but rather from wanting to keep up appearances. It was now clear to me that this had been the pattern throughout our friendship – she hadn't wanted to be Philippa's friend; she'd wanted to be Skinny Latte's friend.

At last, she signed off saying she felt the friendship was beyond repair, with both of us to blame, and it was best we moved on. Taking in her words, bizarrely, I felt the same way I'd felt when my marriage to Glenn had ended: sad because I'd lost someone I had once cared about very deeply, but also overwhelmingly relieved. At the same time, I was ashamed to have carried on with this dishonest situation long after I'd become aware that I no longer trusted Meredith or wanted her in my life. However, I had only been trying to protect myself from more hurt in the only way I knew how. I couldn't keep beating myself up over that.

Meredith actually taught me a lot about friendship. She taught me it's just as important to be happy for your friends when they succeed as it is to be supportive when things aren't going so well. She taught me that sometimes people you care about let you down and there's very little you can do except try to learn something from it. She taught me that holding it together and trying to forgive someone are good things to do, but in the process they can also make you appear far less hurt than you actually are, so the only way through is to be honest.

Most of all, Meredith taught me how important it is to love yourself. I never thought, and still don't think, she is a bad person. She had enormous potential and a gentle heart, both of which got overtaken by her fear of being herself. When you're afraid to be yourself, the only thing that makes you feel good is the approval of others, which you try to get at all costs, even if it means doing something you know at your core is wrong.

For nearly two years, I had believed that my feelings of hurt, disappointment and fury over how Meredith, Gillian and Mel had behaved, and all the crap that was now in my way as a result, was their fault. The truth was, my work with Margot had made me realise, I had blamed those women because it was easier than owning how I had chosen to respond to their behaviour. No one else is responsible for how you feel. That's your job. I'd had every right to my hurt, anger and disappointment, but instead of expressing that at the time and letting myself feel those things, and being honest both with the perpetrators and with the people I knew cared for me who would help me through it, I put on a brave face, kept calm and carried on, which meant the pain was still fresh years later. Whether I like it or not, that was my choice. I'd fallen back into my old pattern – giving responsibility for my emotional wellbeing to other people. Once I understood this, I had to start doing the work again. I had to forgive myself for not handling it as I should have, and move forward.

So that was why I knew I had done the right thing, albeit in the wrong way. While I felt defensive about some of the things Meredith had said, I knew she was right about one thing – the friendship hadn't done either of us any good for years. I was relieved she had called time on it.

I wrote her a short response, acknowledging her message and wishing her well. There was nothing more to say, really. The second I sent it, I felt a release, like something had physically left my body. My colleagues asked me if I'd lost weight. Tom remarked he hadn't seen me this relaxed for years.

At the same time I felt a little frustrated because I knew Meredith would take any opportunity to play the victim, as Glenn had, but I had to trust that any mutual friends who truly cared for me would make up their own minds; the rest I had to let go. But overall, I was pleased I had put someone who had hurt me in her place, that I'd finally honoured the voice inside me telling me to do something about it. I released a hurt rather than continuing to hold myself ransom to it. It felt good.

As the years have passed, I can see that all the changes I had made in my life, and the person I had become because of them, must have been unsettling, maybe even threatening, to people like Meredith who were truly struggling with loving and embracing their real selves. But you can't take responsibility for people feeling hurt simply by you being yourself and trying to live your best life – that's their issue. I also realised that self-esteem and confidence cannot be built solely by surrounding yourself with people who tell you how great you are – those same people may, as it turns out, have a change of heart and decide you're not so great. You *can* choose to love and be proud of yourself, regardless of what other people have to say. So in the end, Meredith and the others taught me one of the hardest but most powerful lessons I've ever learned.

The friend you need most is yourself.

I'll run with you

got back into endurance events in a big way in 2009. I had long
entertained ideas of running a half marathon, despite not
knowing the exact distance of the event! When I did finally
look it up, I wasn't sure I had it in me. However, I had done some
running in the triathlons, and it was the event I seemed to have
the most natural ability for. More importantly, it was the event I
most enjoyed and if there was one thing I had learned about getting fit, it was that if you're not enjoying it, you're probably doing
the wrong activity. Being bored is no excuse for doing nothing!
(Okay, pep talk over.)

After three years at goal, running was still my main way of keeping fit. I measured myself in time rather than in distance, as I didn't
have any fancy watches or gadgets. I used to go out for half an hour.

I didn't really think about what kind of distance I might have covered in that time, but I had built up good aerobic fitness so there was no reason to think I couldn't start pushing myself.

I thought back to those days in the latter half of 2006, when having something tangible to work towards in the form of triathlons had really helped keep me on the straight and narrow, given what else I was dealing with at the time. I needed something similar now, though not quite in the same way. I just needed an outlet. Exercise made me feel fantastic about myself and it kept the mental demons at bay, provided I had the right attitude (which was not using exercise as punishment, but as a way to de-stress, feel good and do something nice for myself).

After building up my distances to over 10 kilometres, I finally had the confidence to register for the UFD Hackney half marathon at the end of the summer. It was intense, but one of the most joyful experiences of my life up to that point. Tom was the most enthusiastic cheer squad. He wore a 'GO PHIL GO' T-shirt he'd had printed especially and it gave me such a boost every time I saw his cheeky grin and proud face on the course. That race, and the training for it, was a real turning point for me. I had taken my fitness to the next level and had actually enjoyed doing so. It made me feel like the low confidence and sadness of the year before was behind me.

Which of course, it wasn't. My counselling with Margot continued and I had to work hard daily on my issues, but the half marathon had done wonders for my confidence. It reminded me I could achieve anything if I set my mind to it. Self-awareness, at least for me, isn't like having a light switched on and then that's it. It's a light I have to keep remembering to switch on. I began to realise it was something I would need to work hard to stay on top of, probably for the rest of my life.

*

In November 2009, Tom and I had returned to London from our trip to Australia, relaxed and happy and filled with love for our family and friends there. London had descended into the greys and mists of the impending winter. One Saturday night, Tom announced he was taking me out to dinner. I was incredibly excited because, given what we had discussed a few weeks earlier in Australia, I suspected what might be coming. He recreated our first date, when we'd gone to Wagamama on the South Bank and walked along the river afterwards ... except this time it wasn't a balmy September evening; it was freezing and pouring with rain. One of the bridges had flooded, so we had to cross at Blackfriars and walk past via St Paul's Cathedral to get to Millennium Bridge, 'our' bridge. It was hardly a slow, romantic walk as it had been the first time. Not wanting to spoil the mood, I gently asked Tom as we power walked hand in hand, brushing wet hair out of our eyes, 'Are you sure you want to do this tonight?'

Tom was adamant, however, and looking back, everything about that night was us – romantic and a little bit insane, but it worked.

We got to Millennium Bridge and the rain had graduated from fat drops to a fine mist. I don't remember how far we walked along it, or whether we could remember the exact spot where he had kissed me for the first time two years ago, but eventually we stopped and Tom dropped to one knee, in a puddle. He brought out the ring he had bought that day, which explained why he wanted to propose straight away: he can never keep a secret! I don't remember if there were other people around – I'm sure there were – I only remember how he looked at me, the nervous smile on his face, the softness in his voice, and not knowing if it was tears or rain on my face. St Paul's sounded out the hour as I said yes, and we stayed there on the bridge, kissing and laughing and looking at the glittery diamond that was now on my finger, until we couldn't stand the cold any longer. We caught a night bus back to Pimlico, managed to find a pub that was still open so we could have a glass of prosecco, and then went home and called all our family and friends in Australia as it was a decent hour there.

It was an incredibly happy and surreal time. Everything about it was so different to what I had experienced before. It was as if saying 'yes' that night had obliterated the last remnants of guilt, shame and sadness about the ending of my first marriage, which made me realise just how much that had been holding my relationship with Tom back. Margot had actually pointed this out to me before. 'The problems in your life aren't what you think they are,' she often said. 'You have to dig a little deeper and be prepared to face yourself.'

Deciding to get married again was a huge leap of faith for me. I was deliriously happy but I was also terrified to a certain degree at first. I felt so grateful to have found this wonderful man, that we shared such a big love, so worthy of celebration, but I also felt I couldn't make a big deal of it because it was my second attempt. But then I realised I was thinking about it way too much. I couldn't worry about people judging me, even though I knew some were. I had to choose my future over my past. I had to follow the advice Dad had given me – to trust what I had with Tom and realise that not only did I deserve the happiness I had found with him but also that everything about my relationship with him was different.

With Glenn it was so obvious (except at the time!) that it was never going to work and yet with Tom, I knew that it would. I was so much more present with him. I loved being with Tom, spending every day with him. I could be myself. Honest communication has always been Tom's modus operandi and therefore complacency and bottling up my feelings were a thing of the past. I also realised that in this marriage I wouldn't be constantly fighting for my dreams and my freedom, as I had the first time, because we actually wanted the same things. I still had my own life, but I also had a shared life with Tom, which made my own all the richer. Yes, there would be compromise occasionally but never sacrifice on the same level I'd experienced before – I'd finally learned the difference between the two. Maybe I still didn't really have a clue about marriage or how to make one work, but I'd found a man who was worth the gamble. I was willing to give it another shot. And that was something, when I recalled the bitter heartache of three and a half years earlier, that I never thought I'd say.

*

Once we had approval to marry from the Home Office (as I was still in the UK on a visa), Tom and I began preparing for our wedding in earnest. I won tickets to a posh bridal fair in Battersea, and I dragged Tom along to it to get some ideas. We entered the conference centre to the sounds of a string quartet playing Seal's 'Kiss from a Rose' and fought our way through the crowds around the stands offering all kinds of wedding-day essentials, from an old-time ice-cream cart for the reception to pearl tiaras (because you get so much wear out of those).

'There's *nothing* here for men,' Tom grumpily pointed out. 'I thought being the groom was kind of important too.' In fact, he was one of the few men there; most of the brides were accompanied by their mothers or friends.

After finding out that hiring the ice-cream cart, the only thing at the fair that caught my interest, was going to cost the amount we had earmarked for the entire reception, Tom and I beat a hasty retreat. We both felt quite depressed as we walked back over the bridge to Pimlico.

'No offence, Phil, but I don't want our wedding to be anything like any of that bullshit,' said Tom. That was a relief, because nor did I! Don't get me wrong – we wanted to have a special day and a lovely party, but the wedding itself was always secondary. I just wanted to be married to Tom. A gorgeous wedding to celebrate your love is wonderful, but it is only one day. I knew that better than anyone.

In the end, we kept things simple. We booked the ceremony at the Old Marylebone Town Hall, a gorgeous gothic building near Baker Street that has hosted many high-profile (but low-key) weddings over the years, including Paul and Linda McCartney's in 1969. Being Beatles fans, we loved that connection and it sealed the deal for us. Wandering happily through Hampstead and Chalk Farm one sunny Saturday in May, we stumbled across a character pub on Haverstock Hill that looked like it was shut for a wedding. We peered inside and saw beautifully decorated tables with flowers, but it wasn't too wedding-y; it just looked like a very tasteful party. We went back when it was open to meet the manager, who gave us drinks on the house and every vegetarian option on their canapé menu to sample. We were utterly charmed, booked the place on the spot and ordered glasses of prosecco to celebrate.

So, we had a ceremony and reception venue. Now all I needed was a dress. I didn't expect to find my 'dream' or 'perfect' dress, I just wanted something pretty, flattering and fun to wear, preferably something I could wear again. Despite going on a mission worthy of an MI6 agent every shopping trip was a disaster and, four weeks out from the big day, I still didn't have a dress. Finally, my old schoolfriend Kristy, who was coming from Hobart for the wedding, came to the rescue and sent me a link to the Etsy shop of a young dressmaker called Eleanor who specialised in 1940s and 1950s vintage styles. She was based in Brighton, a seaside city about ninety minutes out of London, and I called and made arrangements to come to her studio. It was Gay Pride that weekend in Brighton and so the town was jumping, the trains were crowded and all I wanted to do was collapse in a heap. This wasn't how I wanted to spend the lead-up to my wedding to Tom, who had told me over and over that he didn't care what I wore, that I could show up in jeans and a T-shirt and he would still marry me. I felt so shallow for wanting to look wonderful, despite knowing that that's not what it's all about. *If only I could sew,* I thought, *and if only I had more money and if only I was taller and thinner and if only I wasn't such a terrible person for having been married before, because then bad things would stop happening and maybe this is the Universe's way of telling me not to get married ... panic, panic, panic.*

I walked briskly through the buzzing streets of Brighton until

I found the dressmaking studio, where I was greeted by Eleanor and a hot cup of tea.

'I only have four weeks,' I said with trepidation; I'd been turned away from every bespoke dress shop in London when I mentioned that timeframe.

'That's fine,' she replied breezily.

We swept through the racks of beautiful handmade dresses. The one I liked most was made of vintage taffeta in emerald green, with a sweetheart neckline and cut to emphasise the waist. It was beautiful and it fit perfectly – as if it had been waiting for me. Eleanor's studio was in the basement of a vintage store, and we went upstairs into the shop so I could see the dress in the big floor-to-ceiling mirrors. When the girl in the store produced a fluffy 1950s petticoat to go underneath, the whole outfit was transformed and I felt like Marilyn Monroe. Eleanor agreed to make the dress for me with an extra inch on the hem to make it knee-length and give it an air of elegance. I was ecstatic. My search was over.

My parents arrived in mid-August, and Mum and I had a lovely time getting other things organised for the wedding. She helped me find my shoes, earrings and other last-minute things, and she found a flower shop that was closing down and bought all their remaining stock – a mountain of lavender plants, mini bay trees, heart-shaped climbing ivies and some other decorative plants – for the reception for less than twenty pounds.

We all went to Wales for a few days to see Tom's parents and to show my parents a bit more of the UK. I initially thought it was a silly idea to go away just before the wedding when we still had so much to do, but it turned out to be the best thing we could have done. Being out of London, with nothing to organise and being forced to relax, I felt myself unravelling from my tight coil of thoughts. I felt more ready for this wedding and marriage than I had ever felt for anything in my life – something that was definitely missing the first time.

*

Wednesday, 1 September 2010, three years to the day since Tom and I met, a day that might have been like any other were it not for the bizarre coincidences that ensured we were both in the right place at the right time, dawned bright and warm. I woke at about seven and when I pulled back the curtains, happy, golden sunshine spilled in.

It was wonderful getting ready for the wedding that morning. My parents bought a pile of roses from a florist stand at Victoria Station for the bouquets and buttonholes. Hair and make-up started mid-morning, and while the whole beautifying process went on, Dad took the bus to Kensington and brought back a spread for lunch, together with prosecco of course. Everyone made sure I ate something – how very different, I thought, to my first wedding, when I didn't eat anything at all beforehand to make sure my dress would do up. This time, in my gorgeous emerald green gown that did up easily, I felt just how I wanted to feel. Not like a bride, but like the best possible version of myself. Exactly how Tom made (and still makes) me feel.

Just before we left I rang my sisters on Skype, each one in turn, and talked to them for a few minutes. There were a few tears. The only thing I would change about the day would have been to have the three of them there, but two of them were heavily pregnant at the time, so a twenty-four-hour flight was a bit of an ask. As we talked, the wedding photographer snapped away, with me oblivious, so I do in fact have a picture with each of my sisters on my wedding day – me in my wedding finery, them in their pyjamas.

We locked the house, hailed a passing cab, and travelled along in the mid-afternoon sunshine through central London, laughing, chatting, and with me a bundle of joyful nerves. Before I knew it we were through Marble Arch and on Baker Street, heading up towards the Old Marylebone Town Hall. The taxi pulled up outside and I got out of the cab last. There was Tom on the pavement, waiting. I will never forget the way he looked at me, full of love and awe and happiness.

Everyone went into the Blue Marriage Room, where the ceremony was going to take place, and Tom and I went into a little interview room on our own. We held hands, talked softly and laughed, but the longer we waited for the registrar, the more nervous we got. Our ceremony was scheduled for 3.30 p.m. but, apparently, the wedding party for the 3 p.m. slot hadn't yet turned up. (We never found out if they did!) Finally the registrar burst into the room, full of laughs and smiles, and interviewed us briefly. We were then given the go-ahead to come into the marriage room and begin. As we walked into the room, everyone clapped and my eyes swam as I looked around. I barely registered who was there. The room was beautiful, full of fresh flowers (including, my friend Kristy noticed, kangaroo paw, which I thought was a gorgeous touch).

The ceremony began with a welcome and a reading by our friend Ivy, then the moment came for Tom and I to say the vows we had come up with ourselves. I went first. There was so much I wanted to say to him. How do you tell the person who made you believe in love again how much they mean to you? The person you want to give all of yourself to, because you know your heart, your darknesses and your secrets are safe with them? How do you tell them that they make you want to be a better person, to only do good with yourself, as that is what they do? In the end, I think I managed to say all of that, but what I wanted to tell him, more than anything else, was that before I met him, I'd had no idea what real love was.

I could hear quiet sniffles from the audience as I spoke, and to keep my own tears in I squeezed my new husband's hands and looked deep into his eyes, never straying from them. I watched his face soften and break into a grin when I made a joke, felt his hands squeeze mine harder as my voice wavered slightly, and watched his eyes brim with tears as I spoke the last few words.

'How am I going to follow that?' were Tom's first words when it was his turn.

We exchanged the rings, which slipped on easily, as if they had always been there, and signed the registry with David Bowie's 'The Wedding Song' playing in the background. Finally we were presented with the marriage certificate. 'In this country,' said the registrar with a smile, 'the certificate is traditionally given to the woman. Presumably because she needs it to change her name!'

While I wouldn't be doing that, I loved the sentiment. Being handed that envelope was the moment where it hit me: *This really is a brand new start.*

As we went outside we were showered with confetti, posed for pictures in the sunshine, and all the passing buses, cars and taxis hooted their horns and called their congratulations from their wound-down windows. Once we'd had enough of photos, we hailed cabs that drove us up the road to Chalk Farm, where Bellinis and Australian sparkling wine awaited everyone on arrival, as well as delicious vegetarian canapés and bountiful cheese platters with fruit, bread and crackers.

It was the least formal wedding I think I'd ever been to. We had some wonderful speeches from Tom's best man, Ed, Tom's sister, Zoë, and from my dad, who made everyone laugh with his particular brand of Aussie humour and then read a moving speech my sister Liz had written. As the sun set and the fairy lights in the garden were switched on, Tom and I cut the cake and fed pieces to each other, and managed to get around the party to talk to each of the fifty or so guests. Finally we hopped into a cab to take us to Mayfair for the night and then, it was just us. The day had gone so quickly but everything about it had been perfect. I had never felt more relaxed, more loved, more ready for anything. Everything about it had been so different to what I remembered from the first time. This was grown-up and solid; joyful, magical and real. And I knew, finally, that the past was the past. It truly was, as Oscar Wilde put it, the triumph of hope over experience.

Dial M for marathon

our months later, Tom and I were finally leaving for our honeymoon, a full glorious week on the island of Madeira, where we had rented a villa next to the ocean and were looking forward to enjoying some winter sunshine (a popular holiday criterion for UK residents). But this was a honeymoon with a difference – I was now training for the London Marathon. The week before we left, I had received an email from the PR team at Lucozade Sport.

Philippa! We saw your blog and profile in Runner's World. *We have a place for this year's London Marathon on our media VIP team. Would you be interested?*

The London Marathon? *Me?* The most I ever did these days was maybe 5 kilometres after work and that was if I was feeling energetic. I hadn't done a long-distance race since my first half marathon in 2009. I wasn't under any illusions – I was not marathon ready. But I rather liked the idea of finding out what it would entail.

But where on earth would I start? It was already the end of January and the marathon was taking place on 17 April, less than three months away. This would either be one of the best things I'd ever done or one of the stupidest. I hesitated for a while, talking to Tom and my friend and former housemate Louise, now living in the Middle East, who had just run the Dubai Marathon and whose triumph I had enjoyed watching over Facebook. They were both encouraging. My friend Shauna was also just about to launch a new business called Up and Running, an online running school with her friend and professional coach Julia Jones. She had contacted me about helping to spread the word about their program on my blog, which I was of course happy to do. I told them about the offer to run the London Marathon and said I'd appreciate any tips from Julia who, to my surprise and delight, ended up offering to coach me for the whole thing, via email. *You haven't got long, but it can be done*, were her encouraging words. So it seemed, yet again, the only thing standing in my way was me. So later that same day, I told Lucozade, *Yes!*

A week later, I was on my honeymoon in Madeira, running 10 kilometres every morning. I ran along the seafront of Santa Cruz, Lady Gaga blaring in my headphones, all the way out to swimming pools and water parks that had been emptied for the winter, the brightly painted dolphin statues and funfair-like attractions looking eerie and macabre without people around. Afterwards, Tom and I walked to our favourite cafe in the Santa Cruz piazza, the Bom

Jesus, where we ordered coffee and devoured a couple of *pastéis de nata*, the traditional Portuguese custard tarts, which I felt I had well and truly earned.

Returning to London a week later was when it all got real. Coach Julia sent over my training program and I realised what a big commitment this was, for both my body and my lifestyle. I had a full-time job, was trying to write a book and enjoyed a full social life with my new husband. I was going to have to make this work around the non-negotiables, and everything that wasn't essential would have to take a backseat until the marathon was over (a process not dissimilar to the one I followed in the writing of this book).

The thing about taking on a challenge like this is that your life has to adapt to give you the best chance of success. Running after work, for example, wasn't a good idea any more – a breezy 5 kilometres along the Embankment was a lovely way to unwind after a day at the office, but doing three hours of strides and speed work was another thing all together. The only solution was to wake up early and train before work, which meant going to bed early, very much at odds with my night-owl nature. I started setting the alarm for 5.45 a.m., when I would stagger out of bed, half asleep, dress in my gear, drink some Lucozade and head down to Battersea Park to do the regime specified on Coach Julia's schedule. It was freezing cold and dark at first but as February became March, the mornings slowly started getting lighter and the air less bitter. I was trying hard not to be scared of slipping over on icy footpaths, or of the rats darting across the paths and into the bushes. Every morning I ran to the same bench and did my stretches. It helped to have a routine, to go the same way, to do things on autopilot, to think less.

I also had to schedule the consumption of alcohol, which, despite the steely determination of my point-counting days in the past, wasn't easy. Tom and I were typical twenty-something Londoners who worked hard and played hard. It wasn't unheard of for us to unwind at the end of the working day with a gin and tonic. If we went out with friends, it was always 'down to the pub', and whenever I met up with a girlfriend it was usually Kir Royales to start with and then a bottle of chardonnay to share. My writing club even met at a wine bar. Writing all this down I realise it sounds bad, but the honest truth is life was just very social and for me, my husband and friends, that meant having a few drinks. I went to my friend Katie's thirtieth birthday celebrations in Leicester Square a few weeks into training. Tom bought a beer for himself and a sparkling water for me, and Katie's eyes widened. 'Oh my God!' she squealed. 'Are you pregnant?' which of course piqued the interest of the other guests. I got used to similar reactions over the next few months.

I shared my training diaries on the blog and the responses were all very encouraging. I remember feeling, for the most part, overwhelmingly positive. But inwardly I was still a bit terrified. There were horrible runs where I bemoaned my lack of progress, wondering why it wasn't getting easier, or where I had altercations with cyclists who insisted on riding on the pavement instead of the road. On one early-morning run in Fulham a street sweeper backfired in my face and left me looking like Bert the chimney sweep from *Mary Poppins*. But then I had days when it was easier; my body did what it was supposed to do and I got home overjoyed to realise I'd run 20 kilometres before breakfast. Slowly it dawned on me that the reason I was succeeding was because I was disciplined, because

I ran even when it was the last thing I felt like doing. 'That was how I lost those pesky 30-odd kilos five years ago,' I wrote at the time, 'and that's why things are going well now. Getting up to run at 6 a.m. is a drag and I hate it, but this is what I have to do to get what I want. I try not to even think about it any more.'

*

Having lost every weekend for the past three months to training or long-distance races, doing half marathons and 16 mile treks all over the UK and dragging my ever-patient and very proud husband along with me, finally the race I had been running all of the others for was here.

My favourite part about the lead-up to the marathon was sitting around and carb-loading for a few days – although I didn't want to see another piece of pasta for a while – but I found trying to eat breakfast on the morning of the marathon quite an ordeal. Eventually I abandoned the food and just got my kit ready, got dressed, triple-checked everything and then carried my plate and glass through to the kitchen. I drank another orange juice and forced myself to have one more bite of breakfast. Big mistake. No sooner had I swallowed it than I was overwhelmed with nausea. It was time for us to leave but there was no way I could get on the tube feeling like I did. I ran outside to breathe some fresh air and eventually I threw up the orange juice and the last bite of bagel. I felt better instantly. Maybe it was just nerves.

We got the tube to London Bridge and then our overland train to Greenwich, both trains packed with people with race numbers and red bags like me. There were three start waves – the blue, the green and the red, all in different areas of Greenwich, which would merge together after a few miles and then everyone would follow the same course. My red start was in Greenwich Park, which was throbbing with runners, spectators and supporters alike. Tom and I said goodbye at the bottom of the park and then I strode up the hill to the start. It was like being at the circus, with lots of people dressed as animals – rhinos, tigers, giraffes – the smell of grass and tents, and banana peels everywhere! The wait for the loo was quick, to my surprise, and then I went to find a spot in my start zone. There were nine different start zones within the red start, based on the anticipated finishing times we had given the organisers. I was in number 9, among Mr Blobby, a few rhinos, a man with a washing machine on his back and a guy running the whole thing barefoot.

We heard the cannon blast at 9.45 a.m., signalling the official start of the race, and everyone cheered. Then it was a slow shuffle to the start line. I got talking to the girl next to me, who had climbed Sugarloaf Mountain a few weeks earlier as part of her training, and we ended up sticking together for the first 10 miles. We crossed the start line at around 10.10 a.m. and everyone whooped as we went through. I deliberately started out slowly, knowing there were a good five hours of running ahead of me, but I felt fantastic. It was such a happy atmosphere, with everyone in great spirits and chatting to each other, spurring each other on.

Before too long we were out of the park and onto the road, which was lined with local residents cheering us on. The first mile went by very quickly, and the encouraging shouts and calls resounded as we saw the marker. 'Only twenty-five to go!' everyone was saying. I remember thinking, *This will be easy.* By mile 3 we were merging with the blue and green starters but because we were at the back of the red pack I didn't really notice. As we passed the marker for mile 5, I heard a familiar voice calling out, 'Go Phil!' I looked over to my left and there was my friend Lisa! I felt my face explode in a grin. I waved and blew her a kiss and kept going. It's so wonderful to have people you know in the crowd cheering you on. Lots of strangers also called out, 'Good job, Philippa, keep going!' It was such a boost. I was glad I'd put my name on my shirt.

I continued to power on through Greenwich, where the crowds were thick and noisy. With bands playing in the streets, the crowds of people cheering, and some of the runners in funny costumes, the whole atmosphere was like one big carnival. There were even girls running while hula-hooping! It was humbling to watch these incredible people doing some quite difficult and outrageous things, all for a good cause. Equally humbling was seeing pictures of loved ones taped to runners' shirts – children, parents, grandparents, brothers, sisters, friends – the memory of whom was inspiring this gruelling race.

At mile 12 I reached Tower Bridge, one of the highlights of the race, where there was not a spare piece of pavement to be seen – the streets were choked with people, waving banners and shouting encouragement. The atmosphere was electric. I felt quite euphoric to be nearly halfway, and physically I was still feeling great, albeit a little tired. I kept powering on, and at mile 14 I saw my friend Ali, who had come down from Leeds especially, waving and holding a big sign saying, 'RUN PHIL RUN!' I was ready for a little stop, so I bounded over and hugged her, chatted for a few seconds and then off I went again. What a boost!

By mile 15 the road was sticky with gels people had partially eaten and thrown down, the syrupy contents melting in the hot sun. It felt like velcro, and you could hear your shoes sticking and unsticking as you ran. My knees and ankles were starting to hurt at this point as the fatigue started to set in. I had been hoping to get to mile 16 without stopping to walk, but with 11 miles still to go I had to think of the big picture. I wanted to try to run the last 3 miles without stopping, as that was where the biggest crowds were – and hopefully Tom and our friends too – so I had to take a break in order to have the energy later on for the finish I wanted. I kept my eye on my watch and once I'd done five minutes of walking, that was it – I was off again. It was getting very hot and I ran gleefully underneath some showers that were running, enjoying the shock of the cold water on my overheated body. There were lots of barbecues out in the streets, with all the locals making a real day of it, which didn't help my feeling of just wanting to collapse with a cold drink!

I realised someone was slowly jogging up very close to me and looked over. It was Maxi, a girl I had met at a race a few weeks earlier, and who had run most of it with me. What were the odds, in a race of tens of thousands of people? We were overjoyed to see each other again. 'It was fate!' Maxi laughed as we continued along together. We walked for a little bit then ran again at mile 17, which went very fast with a friend to chat to. Eventually she had to stop and walk again, but I kept running. I heard some drums as I veered into Canary Wharf, which was even more crowded than Tower Bridge had been. I was going past the tube station and looked to my left, and there was Tom! I bounded over for a big bear hug, talked to him briefly and then I was off again, calling, 'See you at mile 25!'

I don't remember the next few miles – even writing a race report for my blog the next day I struggled to recall anything about then. I just kept trying to not think about the pain, to keep smiling and doing whatever it took to get through another mile. When I hit the 20 mile mark I remember perking up slightly, as the scenery was starting to look a little more familiar. I saw my friend Ali again when I hit the 22 mile point and thought, *Ooh, only 4 miles to go! That's only two laps of the park! I can do that!*

There was never a point where I didn't think I could keep going. I never hit 'The Wall'. It hurt, yes, but I was expecting it to. I remember telling myself, *One mile at a time,* around this point. It was just before mile 24 that we went into a tunnel, out of the sun, and most people were walking through there, out of the view of the crowds. I had a tiny walk break, just to get some Lucozade into me, and then got running again. I had an enormous surge of adrenaline as we hit the Embankment. I saw the National Theatre, Waterloo Bridge and the London Eye in the distance. I was only 3 miles from my flat. This was my London now. I was sore and exhausted but I couldn't wipe the smile off my face.

I passed Embankment Station and thought sweet nostalgic thoughts about meeting Tom there for our first date. I went under the bridge and then there he was, at the front of the crowd, calling my name. I couldn't stop because I was on a roll, but my eyes filled with tears to see my husband there, smiling and looking so proud. It was just what I needed to see in that moment. He said later how everyone around me looked like they were all about to keel over yet I was grinning like a madwoman and ploughing on. I don't know how I did it. It was just one step at a time at that point.

After passing the marker for 25 miles, I thought about stopping for a minute to walk, just to get enough momentum to do the final mile down Birdcage Walk. But then I saw Big Ben, an image I'd held in mind during my training, for all those months, wondering what it would be like to see it after those 25 gruelling miles. I'm pretty sure it struck three as I approached it. I felt my chin wobble a bit but I didn't stop. I put one aching foot in front of the other. I rounded the corner and saw the street I crossed every day on my walk to work. It was so close now. I kept running with every ounce of strength I could muster. And I couldn't stop smiling.

'You're nearly there!' 'Well done!' came the calls from the crowd. Everyone running or walking around me looked exhausted but well and truly high on endorphins. When we got to Buckingham Palace there was a sign saying, '385 yards to go!'

I rounded the corner to go up The Mall and there was that bright red finish line. I had never been so pleased to see anything in all my life. A sprint finish was out of the question but I kept the pace and threw my arms up with glee as I got closer and ran through. There I was. My marathon was over. Finished. Done.

The sheer elation and awe at what I had just done, when six years earlier I had got out breath climbing stairs, overwhelmed me. It was the proudest moment of my life. I expected to burst into tears but all I felt was pure, unadulterated joy. After receiving my medal and goody bag, I walked through a jam-packed Trafalgar Square, people congratulating me and shaking my hand as I passed them. I finally found Tom and we walked to Leicester Square for the Lucozade after-party, where I got a hero's welcome. I was given a key to a hotel room so I could freshen up. Even though I could barely walk by now, I managed to shower, put on some clean, dry clothes and then we went back to the party for food, drink, a massage and mingling. After a few hours we left the party to have dinner. Tom took me to Wagamama, which was just what I was in the mood for. We had dumplings, edamame beans with heaps of salt, and tofu fried rice, to which I added a lot of soy sauce. I also had my first beer in weeks. To my great surprise I wasn't all that hungry and I was unable to finish either my dinner or my beer. It seemed finishing the marathon had been enough for one day.

We had thought we would get a cab back to Pimlico after dinner, but because the roads were still looking rather chaotic we decided we would walk home. Tom was naturally concerned that I had exerted myself enough, but I was so blissed out and didn't mind a walk at all, and it wasn't far. So we walked through Trafalgar Square and back the way I had come, past the finish line, through St James's Park and over Birdcage Walk, home. It was surreal, seeing this place that had been a hive of activity, a site of triumph and euphoria only hours before, now quiet, folded and put away for another year. Finally we got home, and I got online to find out my official finishing time, which was five hours, nineteen minutes and fifty-seven seconds!

I could not believe that the same girl who had once struggled to run for five minutes had just run a marathon – one of the most iconic races in the world, no less. It had been such an honour. From the moment I stepped into my starting pen, I was surrounded by incredible people – not just my fellow runners doing amazing things for charity or just running to challenge themselves, but the people who showed up to cheer us on; who hosed us down, handed out lollies, played the guitar and the bagpipes, sang, cheered until they were hoarse and clapped until their hands were stinging. The St John Ambulance staff who worked tirelessly to make sure everyone was safe and those who needed help got it. The marshals and the people handing out water and Lucozade at every mile, always smiling. London shone that day. The streets were alive and singing with laughter, support and love. I had never been more proud to call this city my home.

Although I had known the marathon would be hard, I'd also known it would be one of the most joyous experiences of my life. I was determined to have fun and to make it to the end no matter what it took. I wanted to prove to myself, again, that there was nothing I couldn't do if I was prepared to work hard enough for it and believed in myself.

I struggled with all of that at times. But the struggle made getting to the finish line all the sweeter.

Always greener

Life after the marathon wasn't all I thought it would be, much like life after a massive weight loss wasn't either. You are still the same person, albeit profoundly altered by the challenges, goals and events that unfold. Life keeps going and keeps surprising you.

Soon after the marathon, I travelled to India for a work conference. I was in Hyderabad for a few days with colleagues and then travelled solo to Goa and Mumbai for five days. This wonderful trip reinvigorated my love of travel and adventure. Tom and I had also booked a trip home to Australia to have Christmas with my family and meet some new nieces and nephews who had arrived since our last visit. Rather than the usual fortnight, we had decided to go for six weeks and enjoy a bit of the Australian summer. My work had approved some unpaid leave and I was looking forward to some quality time with everybody again.

I was also trying to make my writing a bigger priority than it had been in recent years. I invested in a week-long retreat in Inverness with the Arvon Foundation, a well-known writing organisation in the UK. On that retreat, despite positive feedback from my tutors on the fiction project I was working on, I realised that the story I really wanted to tell was about what I had seen and learned and knew. I put aside the novel I had been writing since 2007 and began a new one, using my own journals as a starting point. It was about an overweight, unhappily married young woman and some significant changes in her life that led to her shifting both the excess weight and the husband. She found herself in – surprise, surprise – Melbourne, slim and single, negotiating the aftermath of her broken marriage. I was essentially writing a memoir but I enjoyed using my imagination to bring some situations I had encountered to far more convenient, or dramatic, conclusions than had been reached in real life! So many people had told me to 'write what you know,' so that's what I was doing. I wasn't sure where it would lead but I was having a lot of fun writing it. Every evening after work, I would walk to 'our' Starbucks in Covent Garden and write on the little netbook Tom had generously bought me for a wedding present, with a chai latte beside me. Tom would join me when he finished work and do some sketching for an hour, before we walked through Trafalgar Square and St James's Park home to Pimlico, hand in hand.

Despite the feeling that I was at last making some real progress with my writing, life in London was becoming difficult. Our rent had gone up and we found, despite still loving Pimlico, that life there had lost its lustre. The flat, once cosy, now felt way too small. I was tired of the noisy neighbours, the constant whirr of suitcase wheels as travellers trundled to and from Victoria Station at all hours, the pigeon poo on the washing, the tramps who smashed our recycling, the meth clinic across the street and various other things I'd always thought of as quirks but that now felt like nuisances.

After a lot of soul-searching and number-crunching, we decided to move out to Tom's bachelor pad, a flat he had bought in his early twenties, in a town called Aylesbury, about 40 miles out of London and 20 miles or so from Oxford. The tenants he'd had in it had broken their lease, leaving the place trashed. We spent what little money we had making the flat liveable again – a fresh coat of paint, new carpets and furniture, as we'd rented furnished flats in our three years together in the centre of the city. It was not impossible to commute to London from this small town – there was a national rail service with a regular timetable, and apparently many people did it. My workplace was happy for me to do two days a week from home and commute in on the other days. Tom had been working hard and was very burned out, so a change was going to hopefully do us both good.

We celebrated our first wedding anniversary in Cornwall, a part of England I had longed to see since arriving, and I wasn't disappointed. I loved the fresh air, sprawling beaches and clotted-cream teas. The quiet and sedate pace of life in the coastal village we stayed in reminded me of where I'd grown up in country Tasmania. The peace and quiet, and how much I enjoyed both those things, reassured me we were doing the right thing leaving London, for a little while at least.

It was a big adjustment, however. We had got used to walking everywhere in Pimlico, with everything we needed a mere ten-minute stroll away at most; even the heaving metropolis of Oxford Street had been barely half an hour away on foot, five minutes if we took the tube. Out in the country it was different, and we were going to need a car, which we couldn't afford for the first couple of months. I hadn't driven for nearly two years and worried I might not even remember how. The days I commuted to London were long, with early starts and late finishes. But Tom cooked (without demanding twenty-four hours' notice) and the house was spotless, so at least I didn't have to worry about that. The days I worked at home were far more relaxed. In fact, life outside of work had become very validating and meaningful for me. My blog, Skinny Latte Strikes Back, was going from strength to strength and had even won a Cosmopolitan Blog Award for best health, diet and fitness blog. This extra layer of visibility was doing wonders for my confidence and many opportunities started coming my way. I was offered a regular column in a running magazine and various endorsement opportunities with big brands, which was all very exciting. The real me, the me I had wanted to be all along but felt I had to put away for the day job, was being celebrated and acknowledged. I was excited. Something had shifted in me and I knew deep down that I couldn't continue to work full-time in my publishing job, but quitting was a scary prospect. Was all this success I was experiencing just in my head? Would I jinx it if I chucked it all in and gave my dream of being a full-time writer a shot? I didn't know. What I was hoping for was to have a peaceful break in Australia, then come back to the UK with some clarity and hopefully go part-time while I tried to make a go of things.

On a Sunday night in November, four weeks before Tom and I were due to travel to Australia, we were sitting with a beer to numb the whole 'do I really have to go to work tomorrow?' feeling. On the packet of crisps we were sharing it said, 'Enter your special code to win a cash prize.' It wasn't a fortune, but I certainly wouldn't turn it down.

'Actually, that's all I'd need,' I said to Tom. 'That would keep us going for a little while so I could finish the book, send it somewhere and get myself started. Let's get online and see if we've won!' But of course, we hadn't. Oh well, I couldn't expect anything to be handed to me, I reasoned. I set the alarm for the morning and went to bed, steeling myself for another week.

A few days later, on a cold but sunny Wednesday, I had commuted in and my blood was dancing with the remnants of my second coffee before 9 a.m. There was a strange feeling in the office. Things had definitely shifted at work recently. I had been with the company since I arrived in London in 2007, steadily working my way up, and it had been the one thing, besides Tom obviously, that had been a constant in my life there. I had put down some roots there; I really liked my colleagues and had many close friends among them. The first three and a half years I had been there had had a glow about them – we were all working hard, certainly, but it was fun, and none of the big bosses seemed all that concerned about our little department. But lately management had been more interested in what we were up to – we were pulling a profit and so it was decided our department would incorporate another that wasn't doing so well. There was a shift in management and a company-wide meeting, with a speech delivered by the CEO herself, who reminded me a little of Margaret Thatcher. She told everyone how well we were doing and yes, a few changes and adjustments had been made, but it was all part of a new and exciting era! It didn't cross my mind to be worried.

That Wednesday morning, my manager tapped me on the shoulder and asked if I had a minute for a chat. We walked together, away from the open-plan office, down a few corridors and towards a meeting room. I had seen a few people led out of the office that morning and it had just occurred to me that none of them had come back. We went into a room where the head of HR and the new director of my department were waiting. They told me that, because of the merging of the two departments, they were restructuring everything and making my job, as well as many others, redundant. I was so shocked, I barely said anything. They handed me an information pack to read over and told me I could go home if I wanted to be alone and take it all in. Normally I'd have loved an excuse to leave early but this was horrible. I was comforted by my manager, who confessed he was just as staggered, and went back to my desk, where thankfully nearly everyone had disappeared except for the people who had received the same news as me. They were gathering up their things, looking like they'd just witnessed a terrible accident.

Like a robot, I grabbed my coat and bag, walked the half-hour to Marylebone Station and took the first train home. I didn't even change my shoes, as I normally would have, and walked the whole way in my heels. I didn't notice the pain in my feet. I felt numb, yet part of me was bubbling with excitement and relief, because the decision to leave had been made for me. But I also felt angry, rejected and ashamed. While I knew the time to move on had been coming, it wasn't how I would have chosen to leave. It reminded me of being dumped. Dumped by someone you weren't crazy about and were thinking of breaking up with yourself, but they beat you to it.

I called Tom on the train and told him the news. He was standing on the platform, pale and worried, when my train pulled in. He hugged me and took me to a nearby pub for a much-needed beer and, because it was one of those posh gastro pubs that were sprouting up all over Buckinghamshire at the time, hot chips with truffle mayonnaise.

While I was grateful there was no king's ransom of a monthly rent to pay in Pimlico any more, and that our living expenses had been curtailed substantially since our move, we were still going to have to keep a roof over our heads somehow. With our extended trip to Australia merely weeks away, applying for jobs now made no sense. What were we going to do? I had a few friends who had been made redundant and they had been given pitiful payouts and had needed to get new jobs immediately. I'd be lucky if I got a month's salary to keep us going.

'Have you looked at the package yet?' Tom asked, noting the manila envelope sticking out of my bag. Actually, no, I hadn't. I ripped it open, read it, then passed it to Tom with a grin on my face.

The figure was what had been on that crisp packet.

*

In many ways, being made redundant from that job was an enormous blessing. It set me free to pursue other options and gave me the financial freedom to do so, at least for a short period. It was a gift – of both time and money – and I was determined to use it well.

I had a lot of 'be sensible' voices in my head, which I knew by now really meant 'I'm terrified' – which, indeed, I was. I was finally going to give this lifelong dream of mine a shot and I was shit-scared that I was going to screw it up somehow, that I would give everything I had and it would not be enough. But there was another voice in the midst of all this chaos, a voice that told me this was all happening as it was meant to and I had to be brave. Most of all, I was tired of not doing what I was put on this earth to do. I was damned if I went another precious year without trying. I wanted to be able to look back on my life and think that even if I hadn't got there, at least I had given it a shot. I stopped making excuses, I stopped letting fear win, and I tried.

My husband was an incredible support and this time made our relationship stronger. But there was a lot of adjustment, for me and for Tom, and there were days when I didn't cope very well. I felt some residual shame and sadness over things ending at my job the way they did. I also knew the odds were stacked against me, with the economy being what it was. There were days when I wondered whether I was really up to the task.

It was another stepping-on-the-scales moment. It was tough, it was scary, but it was also a moment of reckoning. I knew what I had to do and if I wanted it badly enough I'd find a way. It was my choice what happened next.

Beauty and the beast

The United Kingdom was enjoying a very pleasant spell of national pride. Union Jacks hung from telegraph poles, in bunting across hedges and in the windows of every house in our neighbourhood. That summer was one long celebration – first the Queen's Diamond Jubilee and then the amazing London Olympic Games. I watched everything with passionate interest and felt inspired. It was the reawakening of my determined spirit that I had let sink into a bit of a slump over the past few months.

My great plans for life post-redundancy hadn't quite materialised in the ways I had hoped, even though, I felt, I was fulfilling my end of the bargain with the Universe. The year, 2012, had started well enough. On my trip home to Tasmania in January, the local paper had interviewed me and I was blown away by the interest that resulted. A few writer friends had put me in touch with their agents. Everything seemed to be falling into place. Surely this was *it*? I had dreamed for so long of how much fun it would be to work on my book full-time and I woke up every day grateful to be able to do it and tried not to take it for granted. But it proved to be far less glamorous and much more demanding than I thought. I had never worked so hard in my life. And it's not just the writing, rewriting and editing that's tough. Putting yourself out there is tough. Self-promotion is tough. Getting enough nerve to press send on an email to someone you hope will want to publish your work is tough. Fighting your demons, who conveniently appear every time you sit down at your laptop, is tough.

It didn't help that around this time my blog came under attack from a particularly vicious troll. The comments, all left anonymously of course, were deeply personal and cruel, occasionally even bordering on defamation. They were left daily or several times a day for a time, and because they were coming from Australia, they usually appeared overnight or while I was getting ready for bed, times I was never particularly calm or logical. I deleted them and tried to keep a stiff upper lip, but the comments really hurt.

Some people told me I had to expect this sort of thing to happen. You write stuff about your life on the internet, for all to see. And it's popular to boot. What do you expect? I'm afraid I don't buy that, or any of the other rubbish that is flung about in defence of the cruelty that is inflicted upon people who write online. It's bullying, plain and simple. I know I'm not everyone's cup of tea. That's okay. I'd just prefer it if the people who didn't like me, or my writing, simply found another blog to read. Telling people on the receiving end of online abuse to 'ignore it' does nothing – it doesn't mend the hurt, and it doesn't stop the trolls either. I do, however, understand that everything has a dark side, so I had to accept that if I wanted to keep blogging, this was probably going to keep happening. Tom reported the abuse to the troll's internet provider but they did nothing. I started sticking to safe subjects on my blog to try to protect myself. I stopped writing about Tom and my family, as the troll enjoyed attacking them as well. I wrote about food, yoga, running, books, products I was sent to try. I pushed the envelope far less, avoiding anything inflammatory. I realise this was letting the troll win on some level, short of shutting the blog down completely, but I didn't have the strength to fight back at the time. The blog became an easy way for me to write about superficial things, and all the hard, sweaty vulnerable labour was saved for my book. But I was starting to doubt whether I would ever get anywhere with that. The agents and publishers I'd approached about it had been very kind and generous with their feedback, but the answer was always still ultimately no.

I dealt with these blows to my confidence by throwing myself back into activities that had a history of making me feel good and putting various painful experiences into perspective – endurance sport and long-distance running. Writing is not my outlet. It is *an* outlet, but it's not the way I relax. It's how I make sense of the world and as it was now my job, I needed a break from it. I needed reminders that I could stick to something and see it through, that I could set goals and reach them. My friend, the Tasmanian writer Danielle Wood, told me knitting has the same affect on her and the same positive reverberations in her work. We writers need reminding that we aren't the most hopeless people on earth, that we can persevere, we can finish things.

Thanks to the continuing high profile of the blog, I was offered a spot in a trail half marathon in September, taking place in Stonor Park, not far from Henley-on-Thames. (It was also the setting for a scene from the James Bond film *The Living Daylights*, a fact Tom and I didn't register at the time but once we were making our way through the films a few years later, we noticed the scenery looked very familiar!) Trail running is very different to road running. It's more like the cross-country running that I had done at school, with a mixture of terrains: dirt paths, obstacles, varying levels of incline and decline. I love nature and being out in the fresh air so this sounded like a wonderful challenge for me. Near our home in Aylesbury was a lovely nature reserve called Coombe Hill, with views all over the vale, so I trained for this race there over the summer. I ran its rocky dirt paths, hopped over fences, tripped over rabbit holes, and got stung by nettles and covered in mud more times than I care to remember, as it was a wet summer. I loved inhaling the earthy, grassy scents of the woodlands of Coombe Hill; the hay, dust and old wool smell of livestock; even the throat-coating smokiness of the occasional camp fire. On the run home there was a patch of road where the fences were covered in honeysuckle and on a warm morning the smell was so heavenly I would deliberately slow down to inhale deeply. Those aren't the sorts of experiences you get on a treadmill.

Even if you're a seasoned runner on the roads, trail running requires more stamina and endurance than you might expect. And if you're used to feeling quite fit when you run, trail running can be a rude shock. I had never been a speedy runner and yet my slowness on the trails, as I dodged fallen branches and rocks and traversed the dips and peaks of the hilly paths, really surprised me. The lack of tangible progress was discouraging when I was working so hard. The trails, for all their beauty, sucked. And yet there were moments when 'Chariots of Fire' came on my iPod or I stopped and briefly took in the view, the patchwork of yellow rapeseed fields and the vivid green of woods and meadows, and felt the fresh air sweep away my feelings of inadequacy. *It's okay,* I would think. *It's not about being the fastest, the strongest or the one who can run the whole thing without stopping. If you make it to the finish line, that's enough.* Little did I realise how true that would end up being.

The morning of the race, Tom and I arrived at a packed Stonor Park and I stared in awe at all the hardcore runners with their impressive trail gear, compression tights and fluoro knee-high socks. I was in my running capris with a hole in them that I'd patched up with safety pins. We followed the signs uphill to the start, shivering slightly in the chilly early morning mist. The hill was steep – a warning of what was to come. The race was comprised of laps of Stonor Park, each one just under 4.4 miles. The half marathon was three laps, the full marathon six. As we runners gathered at the start, everyone looked really pumped but also a bit apprehensive. I had been warned about 'The Beast', a 90 degree hill that concluded each lap, but I could see lots of hills and wasn't sure which was the one considered to be the most insurmountable.

Finally the starting gun went off and away we went. The start was all downhill and unfortunately, it was all downhill, figuratively speaking, from there for me too. I always say that you won't know if a run is going to be good or bad until you start – but within a few minutes I knew this was going to be tough. My breathing was out of whack and I could feel a stitch bubbling away in my ribcage. I was already at the back of the pack and didn't want to stop and get completely left behind so I kept going, slowly, trying to get my breathing under control. It took most of the first lap to do that because the course was on an almost constant incline. I would try to power up the hills but then when I'd hit the decline on the other side I'd get a stitch almost immediately. I couldn't believe it. I'd run heaps of half marathons before and I had even trained for this race on trails, with hills. I felt overwhelmed with disappointment. I was going to have to walk most of it at this rate and I'd only just started. My pride was forcing me to keep up with the other runners but I knew I wasn't going to be able to do it much longer. I was going to have to forget about everyone else, forget about time, forget about wanting to write a glorious and triumphant race report, and just run my own race. I think that's a good frame of mind to have when you're trying to accomplish anything. I didn't know yet that this race was going to be one of the turning points in my life.

I started feeling better once I was on the last quarter of the first lap; my breathing seemed under control and I had hit a downhill section where I picked up some speed. I thought the start of the second lap must surely not be too far away. And it wasn't – but I had to get up The Beast first. Every runner had stopped to walk up it, which made me feel a bit better, but only marginally, as my legs were burning. I finally made it to the top and went down again for the start of the second lap. At this point, I started feeling less freaked out and more engaged in the surroundings, as they really were beautiful. There was a herd of about twenty wild deer that galloped through the park and were spectacular to watch. I saw Tom, waved and smiled, but as I passed him and had to go up another hill I was thinking, *I can't believe I have to do what I've already done again!* Once the semi-flat beginning of the second lap was over and the constant incline started again, the despondent thinking crept back in and I had to work hard mentally to fight it off. I regularly stopped to stretch my tight calves and found I could run better and for a bit longer after stopping. I had a bottle of Lucozade in my hand which I was sipping at regularly but I still felt a bit empty fuel-wise, so I ripped open my bag of jelly beans and scoffed them down. I should have fuelled more – this was no ordinary half marathon, it was a real endurance race. I wish I had stopped at the energy bar stand at the beginning of each lap but I barely noticed it as I was just so happy to have got to the top and didn't want to lose momentum! Stopping for fuel might have made a big difference.

At the end of my second lap I had just reached the top and was about to start my third and final lap when a marshal got my attention.

'The half marathon finish is over there,' he said, pointing to the left-hand side of the course.

'But I still have another lap to go!' I said, thinking, *Oh dear, I must be very slow if this person thinks I should be finished by now.* I'll be honest – for a split second I thought about going over there and finishing, just so it would be over. Everything was aching, my breathing problems had returned and I couldn't believe there was still more to go. I was so fatigued I was finding it hard to lift my feet properly, which meant I was tripping constantly because the terrain was so uneven. There were rocks and tree roots to dodge, and a lot of the course was on a bit of a slope so one leg had to work harder than the other to keep me upright. I ran for as long as I could and then I would walk to get my breath back and then try to run again, but it was getting harder to sustain any kind of pace for long. I couldn't even run on the flat bits any more at this stage, only the downhill sections. I really didn't think I was going to make it. I was exhausted, in pain and could not understand for the life of me why I was doing this for fun. Mentally I knew I could do the distance but my body had actually started to shut down. Even walking was getting difficult. I didn't remember even the London Marathon being this hard. I felt like such a failure. 'What are you doing here, Phil?' I moaned. And then the P!nk song 'So What' came on my iPod and as I heard her sassy, empowering lyrics, my mind suddenly woke up. The title of that song was the comeback for every negative thought I had.

I'm going to be dead last. SO WHAT?

There's a crowd of marathon supporters coming up and they're going to see me walking and they'll think I'm pathetic. SO WHAT?

Tom is videoing this and I'm going to look fat and ugly! SO WHAT?

I'm going to have to write about how bad this was on the blog and everyone is going to think I suck! SO WHAT? I was going to finish this damn thing, come what may, and if I had to crawl to the finish, so be it.

Finally, The Beast was in full view once more and I knew it was nearly over. I glanced at my watch and saw it was coming up to three hours since the start. That was my worst time ever. I was last, for sure. I wasn't the fastest runner in the world, not by a long shot, but I had never come last in a race. I was flooded with embarrassment, as well as fatigue. Why had I even bothered? Just then I saw a sign on the way up the hill that I hadn't noticed before. It said, 'Dead last is better than didn't finish, and didn't finish is better than didn't start.'

I carried on, through the burn and the all-consuming ache, up that hill. Around me, the battle-weary marathoners were pushing themselves up too. I stopped halfway to catch my breath. One of them stopped with me and then walked up the rest of the hill with me, chatting, telling me he was at the end of his fourth lap. Having someone to talk to really helped. It took my mind off the pain and how much further we had to go, and before I knew it we had reached the top. I thanked him for staying with me and wished him the best of luck with the rest of his race, and then I finally went through the finish line. I had nothing left but I ran anyway.

And then, just like that, the pain was gone. I had done it. I had my timing band cut off, a medal put around my neck, a goody bag and a recovery drink put in my hands, and then I staggered off to find Tom. I lay down in the grass next to him, too exhausted to speak. Tom let me put my sweaty head on his lap and told me he had seen people fall over and keep running with head wounds, or with blooding gushing from various battered limbs. I began to think it had been a miracle I'd crossed the finish line at all.

A few hours later the results were through and I had been right – for the half marathon race, I had come dead last. But, as I'd said to myself for the entire last lap, *so what*? I had still done it. I hadn't given up, even when every part of my body was screaming at me to. I hadn't got injured, which, after hearing what Tom had observed, was an achievement in itself.

I came away from that experience feeling humbler than I had felt in a long time, perhaps ever. Running a race of that magnitude is always an achievement in itself and I had forgotten that. I had succumbed to the allure of the 'after photo' yet again – thinking that just because I had run a marathon before, anything less than that would, and should, be easy for me forever after. I had also put similarly high expectations on myself in other areas of my life – I had won an award for my writing the year before, so surely landing a literary agent and a publication deal would follow pretty quickly? Yet again, it was my expectations that were causing the problem.

Someone has to come last. If we're lucky, it's not always us. But even if it is, it's the price you have to pay for putting yourself out there. For daring to try. For not being in the stand as a mere observer of your life but out in the ring, getting knocked down, fighting to live the best life you can. It takes a lot of guts. And you know I'm not just talking about running any more.

I'm talking about everything. Taking a chance by quitting the terrible job that sucks your soul dry and accepting a pay cut to pursue a career that makes you happy. Moving to another town, another state, another country, because you want to see the world, you want adventure, you want tales to tell, even though it breaks your heart to leave your loved ones behind. Leaving an unhealthy relationship, standing up for your right to happiness. Going to therapy to battle through the things you know are holding you back, to heal your wounds, whatever they might be. Learning to love yourself, despite your flaws and fears. Learning to love your life, regardless of the cards you've been dealt. Trusting yourself, and others, despite being let down before. Forgiving yourself for your past mistakes. Creating something and daring to put it out there, giving it to the world from your heart and soul and saying, 'Here. This is what I have to offer. I showed up and I did the best I could.'

There are all kinds of finishing lines in life. So start running.

Epilogue

When I look at pictures of myself from 2005, I find it hard to believe that was ever me. But I also look at pictures of me taken in 2006, at the dizzy height of my goal triumph, and I can't believe that was ever me either. Perhaps this is just what happens when you get older; you don't recognise your younger self or selves. Or maybe it is because I know I have moved beyond the 'after' photos of 2006 – no longer feeling that what I look like is my greatest achievement or the sole measure of my worth – to a place of greater wisdom and understanding about life and the transient nature of pretty much everything.

In 2005, after I'd stepped on the scales and thrown myself into healthy eating and exercise, all I could think about was what I might look like in a year's time if I stuck to it. I vaguely remembered myself slim and fit, many years prior, but achieving that had always involved a great deal of deprivation. It certainly wasn't something I had done because I cared about myself. The very opposite, in fact.

I had great support from nearly everyone around me – Glenn, Anne, my family, the blogging community – as the kilos dropped and my jeans got looser, but what was overwhelming about the experience was feeling validated for the first time in my life. Sticking to the plan and seeing results made my confidence go sky-high. The more successful I was, the more people noticed. With every scale-related triumph I reported on my blog, the more people came to cheer me on, and the better I felt.

The confidence I had in myself in the immediate aftermath of goal and the year or so after it had been hard-won, certainly, but what I failed to recognise was how much of my motivation was external. What size could I fit into at Sportsgirl? What number did the scales say this week? How many comments did I get on my latest blog post? How many phone numbers did I get while out clubbing at the weekend? Whenever I returned to my hometown, people I had known for years would do a double-take when they saw me or just walk past me all together. I might as well have been a different person, and indeed that was how I thought of myself. I rejected the old me, not realising that the young woman bursting out of plus-size clothes, who got breathless going up stairs and ate two blocks of chocolate in one sitting if she felt lonely, was still there.

The after photo is an ideal so many of us aspire to and yet we don't appreciate it is merely a moment in time. Life keeps going after that picture is taken. It took me years to realise that I couldn't hit the pause button on my life once I'd attained a physical ideal. Life kept going on around me. People changed. I changed. The golden ages sadly don't last forever, as life inevitably moves on to a different phase, but that also means the bad times don't last forever either. Everything is fleeting. You can fight that and spend the rest of your life trying to get back to a moment in time when you supposedly had it all, or you can just make it your priority to feel nourished, happy and fully alive in every moment. You can choose, at any time, how you want to tell your story.

*

I remember the moment I realised why everything had fallen apart so spectacularly and so easily after 2007, when my confidence was in tatters after shutting down the blog and the true nature of some of my friendships was revealed. I interviewed the writer and speaker Nigel Marsh for a podcast in late 2012 and he told me that when we're externally motivated and allow the opinions of others to be paramount in our wellbeing, then our confidence will remain shaky and short-lived, no matter what we achieve. If we are internally motivated, and create change from the inside, it's more likely to be permanent. It was a familiar concept but when I heard Nigel articulate it like that so brilliantly, finally, I got it. I had to truly let go of needing admiration, attention and validation from elsewhere to feel confident and good about myself. I was only going to run a long-distance race if I truly wanted to do it for myself, not to impress others, not to have another tick against my name, not to have something to write about on my blog. Maybe I would see a book with my name on the front cover in a bookstore, maybe I wouldn't. I couldn't hinge my self-esteem on whether or not someone else decided I was worthy any more. I had been faced with this lesson over and over, it seemed, but Nicole in Albuquerque had been right all along. The Universe would keep testing me, to make sure I had learned the lesson. As it turned out, I hadn't. That was why it had all happened the way it had. I couldn't have prevented any of it. I was who I was at the time, doing the best I could with what I knew. Now that I know more, and better, I try to do more. And better.

*

It's now been over ten years since this adventure started, but every day I still have to consciously choose this life. Otherwise it would be so easy to go back to how life was before. But being healthy and fit doesn't mean you live on kale and coconut water. I can put away an entire loaf of sourdough bread on my own and would happily eat cheese and drink red wine every single night. At the end of a long day, presented with the choice of curling up in my armchair to read or going for a run, the chair would always win in an ideal world. But I have to keep myself in check, stay on top of my desire to indulge, and keep myself motivated, because if I don't exercise or eat well I feel like rubbish. Yes, I like my clothes to fit and I prefer not to be breathless going up stairs, but the strongest motivation is feeling strong and alive. That is what keeps me going, what gets me out the door. If I'm feeling a bit unhappy, unmotivated or low, I do a mental recap of how many times I have been running or done yoga recently, whether I've been eating well, whether I've made time to sit quietly and acknowledge what I'm grateful for, or to spend time with people I love. If I come up short then I have my answer. I can't expect to feel amazing if I'm not putting in any effort. You have to pay attention to your life. You have to keep up your end of the bargain. But know that with consistent and focused effort, you really can do just about anything.

*

I haven't run another marathon since the London Marathon in 2011, but the lessons I learned from it continue to reverberate. I feel like it has pretty much prepared me for any goal I ever wish to achieve for the rest of my life. But here's the thing with training for and running a marathon – once you've done it, you know all the rest of your excuses for not doing the things that you dream of doing are just that: excuses. When the rest of 2011 unfolded, and I found myself with a blogging award in one hand and a redundancy package in the other, I knew I had to give my dream a shot. But even though I was acting with love, I was riddled with fear and self-doubt. The book I started writing in 2010 and spent most of 2012 editing and redrafting is the book you are reading now. I originally drafted it as a novel because I still felt too close to a lot of the events. I felt inventing would protect me somehow, and that giving the real events a lick of fictional paint would make the whole story work better. No one would want to hear the truth, surely? I didn't know if I was even ready to face it myself.

But if you want to move forward, you have to face things eventually. It has only been in the retelling of this story that a lot of the lessons over the past ten years have truly sunk in. I've relived all the joy, heartbreak, despair, sadness and euphoria again and I've reconsidered what the events, and the people, were there to teach me. I've processed portions of the tale I'd never allowed much space for in my head, including my own part in them. I acknowledged some of the pain that I was still carrying. I wrote it all out, reading my old diaries and blog entries, trying to entice a story out of all that chaos. Much as my cheeks burned as I relived some of 2006 and 2007, I have a lot of affection for the person I was then. I might not have always made the best decisions, but I was living as fully and as freely as I dared. I was both amazed and frightened of the world I found myself in. I was trusting, hopeful and didn't let go, ultimately, of what I truly wanted. Today I am still all of those things, doing my best with what I know and what I have. I try to show up in the world every day with trust, courage and kindness. I have a voice and I keep using it, however unpleasant the attempts to silence me have been. I am under no illusions that I am at my final destination, or even close to it, but I am committed to my journey, wherever it might take me.

*

I am still floored by how much change came about just from making one small decision that April day in 2005. I'm a profoundly happier woman because of that decision and everything that came after it, painful as it was to negotiate my way through at the time. Since then I've known joy beyond anything I'd ever previously experienced, and I've also been taught things about life I didn't necessarily want to know. The highs have been so high, and the lows have been so low, but life has to have both losses and gains. It took me a long time to accept that. We control freaks don't like life not going our way, but it took me until my thirties before I stopped pushing so hard and decided to enjoy the journey a bit more instead.

Life after 2006, once I'd reached my goal weight and my first marriage fell apart, became about very different goals and a very different kind of journey. I wanted to heal and become my most authentic self – not just because I was convinced my life would be a lot happier, but because I knew it was how I would be of most service in the world. I know that the stories I've told you here are not exactly world peace kind of stuff, but maybe by showing people how important it is to take responsibility for ourselves and our lives, we might be able to tackle the bigger stuff better than we are now? Believe me, no one will thank you for hiding your light and playing small. No one will thank you for not dealing with your baggage. That doesn't serve anyone. The more you fulfil the yearnings of your own heart, the more freely you will give to others. And maybe you'll set off a chain reaction, inspiring others to live their best lives too.

And by best life, I don't mean a perfect life, because I don't know if such a thing exists. We've got to move away from the filters that are all too easy to apply to our lives and embrace everything, including our pasts. It's weird to think that my goal self, grinning at me from 2006 photos, is now a past self, along with the imaginative and bubbly child, the bright but awkward teenager, the hopeful newlywed, the lonely girl in her early twenties, the heartbroken and naive but high-on-life Melbourne girl and the gutsy solo traveller. All of them have melded together to become the woman I am now, who is still learning, still going, still smiling. Letting go of who I thought I was, what I thought I knew and what I thought I wanted was the best thing I ever did.

That's my advice to you, if you're where I was in 2005 or 2006, or even in 2012. Let go. Don't think that because you've screwed up in the past, that means you can't be happy now. You can. Don't think that because you're not in your twenties, like I was when I decided my life had to change, that it's too late for you. It isn't. Open your life, and your heart, to possibilities. Learn to love yourself. All of them. Commit to the journey. Make your choices out of love rather than fear. Trust yourself. Risk being seen for who you really are. Be strong. Go gently and be kind, to yourself and others.

Be careful what you wish for, because you just might get it.

And trust that with every ending in your life, a new beginning is always around the corner.

Acknowledgements

This book owes its existence to the love, generosity and support of many, many people, for whom my gratitude is boundless.

Anne Oettle, to say I owe you a great deal is something of an understatement and without a doubt, my life is brighter, happier, more fun and more meaningful with you in it. Every time I see you, I feel sixteen again. But with some accumulated wisdom, thank God, and without the bad, '90s hair!

Vicky Zimmerman, thank you for introducing me to Becky Thomas, who became my wonderful agent. Becky, if this book were a football team, you'd be the coach. Thank you for everything and for believing in me, even though it took me a while to win a game!

Thank you to Jeanne, Kelly, Imogen and everyone at Black Inc.

and Nero Books in Australia for your guidance, enthusiasm, patience, kindness and juggling Skype dates with me and the UK time difference! Thank you to Sam, Siân and Peter for the beautiful cover.

The editing gods were smiling on me the day they gave me Jo Rosenberg. I feel so lucky to have had her at my side – several continents apart – through this process. From the start I felt she really got me and what I was trying to do. Her touch was gentle yet perceptive and she managed to ask all the right questions to tease the darker, more complicated parts out of the shadows. Thank you, Jo – for making me think, making me smile, and making me own every part of this story.

Thank you to all the readers of Skinny Latte in all its incarnations over the years, especially those who took the time to write to me and share their own stories. There are too many of you to name but you know you are. I am still blown away remembering your kindness, support and friendship. Without all of you, none of this would have happened and this journey might have been very different indeed. I am so grateful.

Thank you John from the Apple store in Covent Garden, London. I told you I'd write a book on that MacBook you sold me! Thank you to the staff at Starbucks St Martin's Lane for letting me sit at 'Craig's table' with my laptop for hours on end.

For a book with a coffee theme, I drank an enormous amount of tea while writing it. Thank you Jacqui, Sally and staff at T2 Tea Shoreditch for bringing a little taste of home to London, and for keeping me stocked in Melbourne Breakfast and Honey Vanilla while I was writing this book.

Thank you Jeanine Stewart for your superb photography, the chats over almond lattes and lemon bars, and for being an all-round goddess of a friend.

Thank you Pat Farmer, Nikki Gemmell and Deborah Conway for all the inspiration over the years and for graciously giving me permission to quote you. George Eliot, I'm still waiting to hear from your people!

Thank you to my kind friends and family all over the world – particularly those who hosted me on my travels. I would especially like to thank Ivy Alvarez, Clare Batten, Brianna Brash-Nyberg, Lisa Cagnacci, Ashley Carr, Alison Clare, Rae Earl, Maryrose Fisher, Emma Holloway, Julia Jones, Zana Khan, Nigel Marsh, Andrea McKibben, Louise Osborne, Katie Parker, Robyn Peel, Sas Petherick, Sunita Ray, Shauna Reid, Paula Rose, Dave Schoon, Julia Schoon, Zoë Schoon, Natalie Seaton-Lucas, Mary Vrjlic, Leonie Wise, Danielle Wood and Sarah Young for being particularly wonderful cheerleaders for The Latte Years. Special thanks to those in the list above who read the earliest and most awful drafts, for your feedback and for spurring me on.

Thank you Andrew Wilcox for all the wine and for being awesome. Thank you Lucinda Mathieson for bringing me Vegemite. Thank you Nicole Emery for everything – next time I see you, I want to give you a big KISS!

Thank you to three very special women – Kristy Booth, Ming-Zhu Hii, Natasha Treloar. If you Google 'balm for the soul', you'll see your names. You've each shared different aspects of this journey with me but you've all been unfailingly kind, patient, enthusiastic, uplifting and wise. Every writer should be so lucky.

Thank you to my wonderful parents, Richard and Sylvia, who must have known early on they were raising a writer and were powerless to stop it. Thank you for buying me books, for reading to me (especially when it was *Dogger* for the thousandth time), for taking me to the library, for being a patient audience at all my early public readings, for putting up with my various flights of fancy and for always encouraging me to dream big. Thank you for always being there and for only ever saying 'I told you so' in a good way. You're my heroes. I owe you everything.

Thank you to my sisters, Elizabeth, Claire and Rebekah – the greatest gifts I've ever got, better than a Dinky Diary or a Barbie Dream House any day – who have shared so much of this journey with me, who have always believed in me, who make me laugh until I cry, and who make me proud beyond words. They say you can't choose your family but my God, I would choose the three of you.

And lastly.

The words 'thank you' don't seem enough for my husband, Tom Schoon, who has supported me through the dizziest highs and the darkest, lowest lows, who put everything on hold to be a lighthouse for me this past year. Bringer of beer, tea or coffee (depending on the hour), he believed in me and this book when it was only a blinking cursor on an empty screen. He has graciously allowed me to share parts of his life and our marriage, and has watched and listened with patience and kindness as I relived every moment of the past ten years. This book is as much his as it is mine. As the Captain and Maria sang in *The Sound of Music*, I must have done something good to deserve you, Tom. You are an extraordinary human being. To thank you for everything you've done for me in the past year alone would take another book. Life with you has been the biggest and most beautiful adventure of all. I'd have you any time.

Lightning Source UK Ltd.
Milton Keynes UK
UKHW04f0836080818
326932UK00001B/188/P